SOUTH AFRICAN WOMEN
LIVING WITH HIV

South African Women Living with HIV

Global Lessons from Local Voices

ANNA AULETTE-ROOT,
FLORETTA BOONZAIER,
AND JUDY AULETTE

INDIANA UNIVERSITY PRESS
Bloomington and Indianapolis

This book is a publication of

Indiana University Press
Office of Scholarly Publishing
Herman B Wells Library 350
1320 E. 10th Street
Bloomington, Indiana 47405 USA

iupress.indiana.edu

Telephone orders   800-842-6796
Fax orders   812-855-7931

© 2014 by Anna Aulette-Root, Floretta Boonzaier, and Judy Aulette

Manufactured in the United States of America

Library of Congress Cataloging-in-Publication Data

Aulette-Root, Anna, author.
    South African women living with HIV : global lessons from local
voices / Anna Aulette-Root, Floretta Boonzaier, and Judy Aulette.
        pages cm
    Includes bibliographical references and index.
    ISBN 978-0-253-01054-4 (cl : alk. paper) — ISBN 978-0-253-
01062-9 (pb : alk. paper) — ISBN 978-0-253-01070-4 (eb) 1. HIV-
positive women—South Africa—Cape Town—Social conditions.
2. Women—South Africa—Cape Town—Social conditions.
3. HIV infections—Social aspects—South Africa—Cape Town.
4. HIV infections—Sex differences—South Africa—Cape Town.
5. Marginality, Social—South Africa—Cape Town. I. Boonzaier,
Floretta, author. II. Aulette, Judy Root, author. III. Title.
    RA643.86.S6A95 2013
    362.19697920082—dc23
                                                          2013018843

1 2 3 4 5 19 18 17 16 15 14

Contents

Acknowledgments

Anna Aulette-Root

When I teach qualitative feminist research methodology to students at the University of Cape Town, I like to emphasize the idea of treating those who participate in research as co-researchers rather than as subjects. In class there is always discussion around the problem of researchers taking credit for studies made possible by anonymous research participants, essentially co-researchers, who because of research ethics must have their identities protected. The problem of the "researcher versus the researched" remains unresolved. The women who participated in the research that is presented in this book were not just participants. Their words, insights, and analyses are what made this work possible. Although their names cannot be listed here or on the cover of the book, it must be acknowledged that fifteen women who live on the outskirts of Cape Town are the major contributors to this book. I would also like to acknowledge and thank the other members and facilitators of the support group, besides those whose stories appear in this book, who contributed their ideas during group discussions.

Thanks to my family, especially my mother and co-author, Judy Aulette. Thank you for supporting me in all ways and affording me the opportunity to participate in the research that is presented in this book. I am grateful for your invaluable knowledge and insight in the field and in the publication process, and, of course, for your huge contributions to this book. I could not have done this without you. Thank you to my father, Albert Aulette, for all of your support and for providing countless hours of grandchild care. Liz Aulette-Root and Olivia Rodbard—thanks to you both for insightful discussions and "life planning." And thanks to my daughter, Azza Aulette-Root-Toyer, for allowing me to sit long hours at the computer and for trying hard to be good.

My supervisor, mentor, and co-author, Floretta Boonzaier—I thank you for taking me on as a student when we met in 2005. Your supervision and friendship have been instrumental in helping me shape ideas into a research project that is meaningful. Thank you for your collaboration in this book, and thank you for the knowledge and opportunities you have offered to me.

My brilliant friends and colleagues in the Men, Masculinities & Violence research project at the University of Cape Town have been hugely important in enabling various research projects, including this book. Taryn van Niekerk, Jacque Matthews Mthembu, and Kim de la Harpe—I am lucky to have friends like all of you. Thanks for all the advice, favors, intellectual discussions, jokes, and thanks for letting me rely on you.

Floretta Boonzaier

I would like to reiterate acknowledgments to everyone Anna has mentioned. Most of all, I would like to thank Anna for her hard work and dedication in bringing this book to fruition. Working with you continues to be a pleasure. I am also grateful to Judy, whose input has significantly strengthened the work. I look forward to continuing collaborations.

Judy Aulette

In addition to all of the people Anna has acknowledged as essential to this project, I also thank Anna and Floretta for inviting me to participate in this project. I am grateful to Floretta for her knowledge of the field and her skill in research methods and analysis. I thank Anna for her creativity and tenacity in developing the original ideas and following them through to the final work. And I am especially proud of Anna as a colleague, a co-author, and my daughter.

From all the authors

Thank you to Dee Mortensen and her staff at Indiana University Press for taking an interest in and being patient with our manuscript. And thank you to Mark Hunter, author of *Love in the Time of AIDS: Inequity, Gender, and Rights in South Africa,* for all of your helpful insights and suggestions in your review of our manuscript.

SOUTH AFRICAN WOMEN
LIVING with HIV

1   Women Living with HIV

This BOOK IS about women living on the margins. Already pushed to the edges by systems of inequality and oppression through global politics, social class, racism, and gender injustice, they are forced even further from the center by their HIV-positive status. This book is also about women who have devised strategies to bring themselves back to "normal" and to challenge what is considered normal. The women whose voices we hear in the text are living with HIV in Cape Town, South Africa, an area hard hit by the HIV pandemic. By listening to their stories we are made aware of new ways to think about HIV, and, most importantly, we learn lessons that are essential for understanding HIV and determining effective routes to its demise.

HIV Is a Social Issue

At the February 2010 annual meeting of the American Association for the Advancement of Science (AAAS) in San Diego, research fellow Dr. Brian Williams, of the South African Centre for Epidemiological Modeling and Analysis in Cape Town, announced that if we could aggressively distribute antiretroviral medicines (ARVs) to everyone who is HIV positive, we could stop the virus from spreading and eventually eliminate it from the globe. ARVs reduce the viral load, the amount of HIV detectable in blood, so dramatically that those who are HIV positive become nearly noninfectious (BBC, 2010). This is a bold and apparently valid idea, but it is a goal that cannot be met if we do not take into consideration the social and political character of the human community, perhaps especially the factor of gender injustice.

The women in this book identify the social issues that go hand in hand with Williams's proposal. They tell us what also must be done in collaboration with the medical breakthroughs. From them we learn, once again, that humans are social and that the complex and contradictory web of relationships and social arrangements in which we live our lives is not easily infused with medical breakthroughs. If we are to eliminate HIV, we must pay attention to a vast array of concerns, including gender, intimate relationships, poverty, stigma, paid work, racism, care work, interpersonal violence, and body aesthetics.

Listening to marginalized women opens up a whole new (and large) box of issues to consider. Our next step must be to bring these margins to the center. We need to place real peoples' experiences and ideas at the center of our thinking about policies and strategies for addressing HIV—not only in Cape Town but in all corners of the world.

The HIV Pandemic

The origin of HIV is a subject of great controversy. Even the date of when it first emerged is unknown, but physicians began to recognize and diagnose the virus among large populations in the early 1980s (Avert, 2010a). For the past thirty years, HIV has expanded rapidly throughout the world, affecting people in all nations and in all walks of life. The spread of HIV, however, has not been uniform. Some populations are significantly more vulnerable than others. The pandemic "is fuelled by the forces of inequality, social exclusion, and economic vulnerability" (Piot, 2001, p. 609). Sub-Saharan Africa is one area of the world where these kinds of inequities and injustices are rampant, and thus the region reportedly has the greatest proportion of people living with HIV. By 2011 an estimated 23.5 million people in the region were living with HIV (UNAIDS, 2012b).

In addition to affecting most significantly those people in the poorest regions of the world, HIV disproportionately infects those who are most vulnerable to inequality, social exclusion, and economic challenges within national populations and communities. Gender injustice places women in a position of less power and greater poverty in all nations. Not surprisingly, gender is a crucial factor related to HIV, and women increasingly make up one category of those most likely to become HIV positive (UNAIDS, 2008). While the virus is a serious public health problem regardless of gender, gender inequities are increasingly making HIV especially devastating for women. In South Africa, for example, 20 percent of women between the ages of 15 and 49 are HIV positive (Statistics South Africa, 2011). Twenty-eight percent of women ages 25–29 are HIV positive, and "HIV disease" ranks in the top ten causes of death for both South African women and men (Statistics South Africa, 2011). Globally, women and men are about equally likely to be HIV positive, but in the areas hardest hit by the virus, women are now the majority; for example, 59 percent of the adults infected with HIV in sub-Saharan Africa are women (UNAIDS, 2011). In addition, the speed at which HIV is infecting people is faster among women than among men. We can, therefore, expect the gender gap in HIV to continue to grow all over the world.

As the HIV pandemic has unfolded, international, national, and local organizations have expanded their efforts to support people who are HIV positive in order to stop the spread of the virus and to diminish the health problems for those who are already living with it. As the presence of the virus escalates in most parts of the world, and for women in particular, it is increasingly imperative for women to receive the most effective social and psychological support possible in order to facilitate improvements in their own health and to safeguard the community from worsening conditions that result from the spread of HIV.

The research reported in this book explores the specific character of gender that shapes women's experiences of living with HIV. What does it mean in the real lives of low-income women in South Africa to say that "forces of inequality, social exclusion, and economic vulnerability fuel the epidemic"? How do gender inequality and the oppression of women affect poor women living with HIV? And how does the organization of gender stand in the way of women protecting themselves from infection as well as prevent them from caring effectively for themselves if they are already infected?

Putting Politics into HIV

The crisis of HIV has been widely reported in regard to some aspects, but remarkably limited research has been done on the problem as it relates to social and political causes and consequences in the lives of women living with the virus. The most important limitation of current research is the narrow perspective that frames much of the work. Most of the existing research has been generated within the confines of seeing and treating HIV either as a matter of bad choices by individuals or as a biomedical problem that can best be combated through education about making safer life choices or through intervention by the scientific community's development of medication and preventive vaccines. The dominant view has paid less attention to the social and political character of HIV. Although it is useful to distribute health education materials and continue to try to find medical solutions, if HIV is a problem that is exacerbated by inequality, social exclusion, and economic vulnerability, these social factors must be put front and center if we are to successfully eliminate the virus. Indeed, the efficacy of education and medical approaches are undoubtedly hindered by social and political barriers, and if inequality and injustice are not addressed, even the best medical and educational interventions will flounder.

The ongoing debate over the distribution of ARVs illustrates the kinds of political barriers that must be overcome in order to address HIV. ARVs are the medicines that have been developed to suppress the HI virus, with India being the largest exporter of generic ARVs in the world. Because its legal system requires more stringent rules than most countries to qualify a drug for a patent coupled with its manufacturing capability, India produces about 80 percent of all generic drugs delivered by donors to people in low- and middle-income countries.

A generic drug is an identical copy of a brand-name drug. Generics are exactly the same as their branded counterparts in dosage form, safety, strength, route of administration, quality, performance characteristics, and intended use. The notable difference between brand-name drugs and their generics is the price (Avert, 2010b). The distribution of generics delivers much lower priced drugs and in doing so brings down the price of brand-name drugs. For example, the most common ARV sold in 2000 cost more than $10,000 annually per patient. Generic

ARVs, which cost about $350 per patient annually, were introduced to the market in 2001.

In the past decade, the multinational pharmaceutical company Novartis has taken legal action against the Indian government for its distribution of generic ARVs. Novartis maintains that it has lost profits due to what they argue is the unfair practice of selling less-expensive generics. Novartis demanded that the Indian government forbid those pharmaceutical companies that were producing generics from continuing their production (Oxfam, 2007, August), but the Indian courts ruled against the company's request to patent drugs in this case. Indian justices argued that granting a patent would make essential drugs inaccessible for millions of people who cannot afford to buy the brand-name drugs and who therefore rely on the generics. After the ruling against the company, Novartis chose not to pursue the action for this particular form of HIV medication. This legal decision has been hailed as an important success for HIV-positive people, but it applied to only one particular ARV medication. The system of for-profit development and distribution of drugs coupled with legal structures that support the rights of pharmaceutical corporations continues to remain in place.

"Customers" who have few resources will continue to face the problem of inaccessible medications with each new cycle of the development of ARV drugs. As each new and more effective treatment is developed and introduced to the market, it will be sold at the highest price the market will bear. This makes medications inaccessible to those who cannot pay until each drug is developed as a generic and then moved through the legal process of defending in the courts their right to distribution. Today most people are still being treated with first-line drugs that are available as generics, but increasingly they are becoming resistant to the first-line drugs and are in need of the second line of treatments, which are being contested in patent cases (Avert, 2010b).

The issue of generic ARVs is only one example of political barriers to getting biomedical solutions to those who need them. Even when generic ARVs are available from global companies, delivering them to those who need the treatment often fails. This is the challenge the Treatment Action Campaign (TAC), an activist organization in South Africa, has undertaken (TAC.org.za). The TAC was founded in 1998 in Cape Town to advocate for increased access to treatment, care, and support services for people living with HIV. For more than a decade it has held the South African government accountable for HIV service delivery. In addition, the TAC has vigorously campaigned against AIDS denial. For many years, some government officials at the very highest level denied the fact that HIV was the virus causing AIDS and furthermore refused to accept that ARVs were the best treatment available for addressing the problem. By staging a huge civil disobedience campaign, the TAC was able to bring enough public pressure on the government to make the South African cabinet overrule President Thabo Mbeki's block of an ARV roll-out program. As a result, ARVs began to be distributed across the country. The TAC was also instrumental in making the government establish a country-wide mother-to-child-transmission program providing ARVs to pregnant women so that the virus would not be passed on to their newborns. In addition, the TAC has challenged multinational pharmaceuticals to make treatment affordable. The TAC's constitution asserts that they will continue these efforts to "challenge by means of litigation, lobbying, advocacy, and all forms of legitimate social mobilization, any barrier or obstacle, including unfair discrimination, that limits access to treatment for HIV/AIDS in the private and public sector" (TAC, 2007, p. 5).

Technical medical solutions are not enough if political, economic, and social barriers prevent people from obtaining access to the medicines science has created. As long as our economic structures demand that stockholders reap huge profits from their investments in pharmaceutical companies and legal systems protect the rights of stockholders over the rights of those who need the medicines, we will be unable to solve the HIV problem. As long as governments deny that HIV is affecting their citizens or hesitate to develop programs to support people living with HIV, we remain a long way from eliminating HIV.

But economic and legal structures are not our only problems. The disproportionate rate at which women are being infected with HIV reveals another political system—gender injustice—which also plays a role in the progression of the epidemic. Gender coupled with economic inequality creates a powerful force standing in the way of winning the battle against HIV.

Learning Our ABCs

Since the discovery of HIV, activists and political leaders have wrestled with the challenge of developing effective programs and policies to address the problem. Most are convinced that education is an essential, perhaps the most essential, tool we have to combat the virus. Much of the approach and materials for HIV education has centered on the concept of ABCs: Abstain, Be faithful, and use Condoms. At first glance this advice appears to be sound. Increasingly, however, those who are familiar with gender-equity issues are asserting that the ABCs fall far short of being effective in women's lives; they may be a valid goal, but for most women they are impossible to meet. Much deeper and more difficult problems will need to be tackled before women are able to protect themselves from infection by HIV (Booth, 2004).

Abstinence is one of the ABCs. Abstaining from sex, however, is not realistic for most women. Abstinence is difficult for nearly all humans, including females. Powerful emotional and physical urges cause women to seek sexual intimacy. But even if we set aside those drives coming from within women, most women do not have control over their sexual encounters because of forces beyond themselves. They may be victims of rape, or they may be partners in marriages where they are legally or morally bound or coerced into maintaining sexual relationships with their husbands. Women may also be required, or at least encouraged, to bear children and ostracized if they do not do so. In addition, a woman's own desire for children presents another significant barrier to abstinence.

Being faithful is another component of the ABCs. However, even if women are monogamous with one partner, their fidelity has no bearing on the sexual activities of their partner. We are now increasingly aware that for many men, the successful attainment of masculinity involves having multiple sexual partners. Being faithful is an empty solution if one is faithful to a man who has multiple partners himself. Ironically, being faithful to a man who is sexually engaged with many others or who is HIV positive is riskier than being unfaithful and taking a partner who has fewer other partners or who is not HIV positive.

Using condoms is the third rule of the ABCs. This solution is a valid one, but it too is largely out of the hands of women. When we use the word "condom" we most often are speaking of male condoms, and the millions of packets of condoms that are distributed around the world are nearly all for male bodies. Women may threaten or cajole men to use male condoms, but ultimately it is the choice of the male partner as to whether he will wear a condom or not. Female condoms are more difficult to find and use, are more expensive, and demand a willing partner in order to use them successfully. Furthermore, ideologies and emotions related to love may contradict condom use for both women and men when they believe that loving means sexual relations unencumbered by preparation and protection from disease (Cole & Thomas, 2009; Hunter, 2010; Preston-Whyte, 2000).

All three of the ABCs are mostly beyond the control of the majority of women. Underlying women's lack of control over these three factors is a much bigger and more potent one that has largely been ignored, and that is the factor of gender injustice and the unequal distribution of power among women and men. Women in virtually all existing societies and in nearly all relationships have less power than men. The efficacy of the ABCs is premised on the degree of control that individuals have over their lives and their sexual encounters. But women often have little control over their own sex lives and even less over the sex lives of their partners. The ABCs, therefore, do not work. And their ineffectiveness points to the question of gender relations and gender politics as the key to finding real solutions to HIV.

Scholars are beginning to question the ABCs, suggesting that three more letters needed to be added to our efforts to eliminate the virus: GEM. Dworkin and Erhardt (2007) propose that our strategies must include: Gender relations, Economic contexts, and Migration (GEM). They write: "In the third decade of the epidemic, it remains vital to not just emphasize how individuals need to change and maintain their own behaviors. Rather, we must also emphasize how successful prevention strategies need to take into account gender relations, other relations of social inequality, economic contexts, and migration movements" (p. 15).

Dworkin and Erhardt argue that all of these are political and economic questions that must be central to our solutions. These issues of power are evident in women who are not HIV positive and are attempting to remain so. They are also evident—perhaps even more evident—in the lives of women who are already living with HIV and are struggling to take care of their health and to prevent the further spread of the virus. This book supports the view of Dworkin and Erhardt (2007) and others who take a political view of HIV as we attempt to uncover the specifics of what precisely needs to be addressed in our relationships of power in order to halt the virus.

What exactly is women's experience with HIV? What does it mean to say that women need power not only to prevent themselves from being infected but also to take care of themselves if they do become infected and to help them prevent the spread of HIV to others? What issues of power have emerged in women's lives as they live with HIV? What are they trying to do, and what stands in their way? In particular, how do stigma, gender inequity, poverty, and violence create barriers to living healthy lives, and what have the women done to try to manage or confront these barriers? This book addresses these questions by exploring the experience of HIV-positive women in Cape Town, South Africa.

Frameworks for Exploration

The research reported in this book addressing these questions is framed by critical postcolonial feminist theory and qualitative methodology. Critical feminist theorists maintain that the world is not the same for women as it is for men. Gender creates differences in their experience, and critical feminists argue that gender is not a system of separate but equal. Rather, social relationships and social institutions place women in subordinate positions (DeVault, 1999). Feminists assert that gender inequity and injustice make it essential that we listen to the voices of women living with HIV in order to ensure that we have the information essential to effectively tackle the problems women face.

The qualitative work we present is situated within the discipline of psychology. Traditionally, psychological research is a field in which men and a masculine point of view have dominated. According to Boonzaier and Shefer (2006), psychological research has been "largely carried out by men, on men and for men's benefit" (p. 8). Feminist research seeks to address this imbalance and is characterized by several principles. Feminist researchers strive to: (1) bring the voices of marginalized people back into the theory; (2) conduct research that has political implications that may lead to positive change; and (3) pay close attention to and attempt to minimize power imbalances between themselves and the people participating in the research (Boonzaier & Shefer, 2006).

Postcolonial theorists assert, furthermore, that when it comes to understanding women, one size does not fit all. Postcolonial feminists "focus on the world's division of nations into so-called First World nations (heavily industrialized and market-based nations located primarily in the Northern hemisphere) on the one hand and so-called Third World nations (economically developing nations located primarily in the Southern hemisphere) on the other" (Tong, 2009, p. 215). The history of colonialism and the contemporary relations of power between those nations of the Global North and those of the South have created a social world that demands that we look at gender only as it is related to global inequity.

"Postcolonial feminists argue that it is essential we develop a radical, anti-imperialist feminism anchored in a politics of dissent for both our theoretical inquiry and the practice that must be linked to that theory" (Mohanty, 2006, p. 7). This statement by Chandra Mohanty, a noted postcolonial feminist theorist, has several components. It asserts that feminists must be radical—that is, they must challenge the status quo by critically assessing the widely accepted ways of thinking and acting that sometimes make "business as usual" appear to be normal and inevitable.

Mohanty also points out that feminists should be anti-imperialists, confronting not only the inequities that exist between women and men but also those that persist between nations. She uses the term "imperialism," which is the classic concept for describing the unequal and exploitative relationship between powerful wealthy nations and the people and nations they control politically and economically. Angela Gillian (1991) explains that according to postcolonial feminists, "the separation of sexism from the political, economic, and racial is a strategy of elites. As such, it becomes a tool to confuse the real issues around which most of the world's women struggle" (p. 229).

Mohanty's definition also includes the requirement that feminists link theory and practice. She insists that our scholarly work should develop better ways to think about the world—that is, theories. Our work, however, must also develop better ways to act on the problems we uncover and explore. It is not enough to interpret the world; we must also change it (Marx & Engels, 1848/2007). Applying Mohanty's ideas to our research requires us to find effective applications for our work in order to uncover how social change activists, such as HIV support group facilitators and members and ARV program facilitators, can help to modify those power relationships, thereby decreasing women's exposure to HIV. Our goal is to ensure that the findings are useful to women who wish to successfully participate in programs that help them to more effectively maintain their own physical health, decrease the development of resistant strains of HIV, and preserve their human rights.

While all of these principles were part of our study, the most important feature affecting the methods we used in our research is the notion of bringing back marginalized voices, or replacing the "view from above" with the "view from below" (Mies, 1983). This practice allows us to study, understand, and amplify the voices of people who have historically been "ignored, censored or suppressed" (DeVault, 1999, p. 30)—in this case, specifically, Coloured (the use of this term is explained in chapter 2) South African women who are HIV positive and living in impoverished conditions in a nation of the Global South.

In addition to being framed by a feminist perspective, our study is distinguished by the qualitative methods that we used to explore the issues. "Qualitative research is naturalistic, holistic and inductive" (Terre Blanche, Durrheim & Painter, 1999, p. 43). An inductive qualitative approach is required if the purpose of a study is to explore phenomena that are interrelated as they unfurl in real-world situations. In light of the body of literature surrounding gender and HIV, the contextual issues in the lives and experiences, along with the medical, psychological, or social problems of women who are living with HIV, are sensitive, complicated, and interrelated. They are therefore best studied using a qualitative approach.

Qualitative research also has another key advantage. It is better than quantitative methodologies at uncovering what might be called the inside story, because it shifts control of the questions from the researcher to the researched. Quantitative researchers, for example, usually create questionnaires with answers from which participants must choose, thus restricting how the questions may be answered. Qualitative researchers may begin with preconceived questions, but they are open-ended, which allows for the logic and concerns of the participants to emerge as they explore the issues. Qualitative methods allow us to ask more directly: what do those people most profoundly affected by a social question have to say about it? Nancy Naples asserts that in too many cases this question is not addressed and that those people who are directly affected by social issues are positioned as dependent others whose needs are determined by the "experts." We must all work to address the needs of women who are HIV positive, but first we must know what the women have determined those needs to be (Naples, 1987).

Much that has been written about HIV, however, is from the perspectives of scholars and medical authorities. There appears to be a gap in the HIV literature when it comes to hearing the voices of women who are living with the virus and their ways of defining themselves and interpreting their own lives. Professionals tell us that the experiences of women living with HIV are complicated by a number of issues, including medical and social constructions of the "disease," interpersonal relationships, and gender dynamics. If we wish to know how all of these complications play out in women's lives and want to hear this information from the women themselves, a qualitative approach is essential. Indeed the discoveries in our research come from the women who participated in the interviews by sharing their perspective, and as we shall see, their insights were often quite different from those that dominate the discourse on HIV among scholars, policy makers, and the medical profession.

Road Map to the Book

This book begins with a description of the social terrain of marginalized women in South Africa. Boasting the oldest human populations in the world and (almost) the newest constitution, South Africa has a long and extraordinary history of ancient human cultures, slavery, colonialism, apartheid, and revolution and now finds itself on the world stage as a leader among nations. But South Africa remains a nation with much work to accomplish in order to make it a just and bountiful place to live for all of its residents. It also remains a nation with a profound public health problem of continued high rates of HIV. At the same time, it is being held captive by global economic forces—in particular, debt and poverty.

Chapter 2 relates some of this history and the contemporary context that frames the lives of the women whose stories are at the heart of this book. The chapter also specifies the particular population group or racial ethnic community within South Africa that has been especially hard hit by HIV and from which the women in our study come. Chapter 3 introduces the support group in which the women met and explains our participation and the methods we used in the study. The fourth chapter focuses on the issue of HIV stigma and the multiple forces of marginalization of women living with the virus. Chapters 5 through 9 report the experiences and responses of the women in our study. The fifth chapter explores the problem of disclosure and the multiple ways women negotiate this difficult challenge with employers, family members, and strangers. Chapter 6 reviews the process of normalization through work activities and relationships with men, including the experience and expression of love in heterosexual relationships. Chapter 7 explores the issue of care work by looking at the overall connections among care work, gender, and HIV and some of the specific ways these connections are reflected in women's relationships with their children. The burden of care work is especially salient for women when it is done in the context of violent encounters with the men in their lives, and this is the topic of Chapter 8. Chapter 9 explores the clash between the need to take antiretrovirals and the problems such drugs cause in altering women's bodies in ways that they find run counter to gendered expectations about women's appearances. In the final chapter we pull all of the strands together to investigate how these issues both shape and are shaped by ideas about what it is to be a woman. Chapter 10 concludes by reviewing the alternative discourse about HIV offered by the women in our study and examining how the social construction of femininity appears as both a source of their problems and a tool for attempting to cope with or confront the problems they face as people living with HIV.

2 The Cape Coloured Community

THIS BOOK IS about women who face stigma, discrimination, poverty, and violence. It is about women who do care work for children and men, and whose responsibilities sometimes force them to make choices between their own needs and those for whom they are caring. And it is about women who must contend with all of these challenges at the same time they fear for the deterioration of their own physical selves and their lost beauty as a result of HIV. Women all over the world face similar challenges, and in that sense the women in our study represent the experience of women across many borders. The women in this case, however, also represent one particular community on the globe with its own unique history and its own particular expectations about women. This case study is about Coloured women in Cape Town, South Africa. Who are these women?

In the United States the word "colored" is an offensive holdover from the period in American history when apartheid was legal under Jim Crow laws. In South Africa, however, while there is controversy surrounding the language used to describe various groups of people in the country, the term "Coloured" is generally not perceived as a derogatory term. In fact, it is widely used by people who identify themselves as Coloured. The identity of Coloured and the character and experience of the Coloured community is an important feature of South Africa to be explored. And as our research unfolded it became an essential issue for discussion in order to understand the lives of women in the Western Cape who identify themselves as Coloured. This chapter describes a little of the history of Coloured people through slavery, colonialism, apartheid, and the struggle that finally toppled a racially defined government in the 1990s. It also provides some context for understanding contemporary issues in the Coloured community as South Africans continue the fight to depose the deeply entrenched social, economic, and political remnants of that history and as Coloured women face all of these issues in addition to gender injustice.

Oldest Humans, Newest Constitution

South Africans like to point out that their history is long. The Cradle of Humankind, near Johannesburg in the middle of the country, is perhaps the earliest site of humans using fire. In 1997 the oldest footprints of a modern human ancestor, believed to have been made 117,000 years ago, were discovered fossilized in the sand north of Cape Town (Beck, 2000). Scientists in 2010 announced that a locality on the southern coast of South Africa, Mossel Bay, "may have been the original location for the lineage that leads to all modern humans" (Brown et al., 2009, p. 861).

Much of this nearly 200,000-year history has been lost, and our summary here reflects the dominance of the European point of view, which makes vast areas of the globe and huge populations of people invisible. We try in this chapter to bring in as much information as we could find about the different populations groups who have lived in South Africa, but the sources and information that have been documented and saved are largely from a European point of view and focus on the activities and experiences of the colonial people who began coming to South Africa 500 years ago. Nevertheless, some information can be gleaned from the history of the encounters of colonial populations with the people they found in South Africa, including those who were there first.

South Africa's indigenous population, now called Khoisan, have been living in South Africa as hunter-gatherers and fisherfolk for tens of thousands of years. The San people were primarily hunter-gatherers, and the Khoikhoi were herders and fisherfolk. Estimates of the precolonial population of San range between 150,000 and 300,000 in the whole region of southern Africa, and between 15,000 and 50,000 in the southwestern Cape. About 200,000 Khoikhoi lived in the area. Their numbers, however, were decimated by genocidal colonial policies and the practice of colonial farmers who took over land and water, leaving the San no place to forage and the Khoikhoi no place to tend their animals and farms. Today the two names have been collapsed into the term "Khoisan" to describe all of the original people in southern Africa (Adhikari, 2011).

Before the arrival of the colonial powers a few thousand years ago, various other groups of people traveled down the continent to settle and establish Zulu, Xhosa, and other population groups in the southernmost region of Africa. By the sixteenth century European explorers had landed briefly on the shores, and in the mid-seventeenth century the Dutch and English began to settle along the coast.

The shortage of labor and the enormous economic opportunities for cultivating the land, raising cattle and sheep, and, eventually, mining minerals (gold and diamonds) led the European settlers to look to the local San and Khoikhoi people for labor. The first records of Europeans taking San people captive to work as slaves date back to 1715. Colonists carried out organized genocidal attacks, destroying the environment where San people foraged, barring them access to water sources, shooting San men, and taking children and women hostage to labor as slaves. Although settlers were prevented from buying and selling people they had captured, in every other way the captives were in fact slaves, restricted from leaving their captors, subjected to unremunerated hard labor, and provided no protection from arbitrary brutal treatment by masters (Adhikari, 2011).

Commandos of colonial men were organized to carry out annual raids on San people in late winter and early spring when farmwork was quiet and the weather was cold enough to require San groups to set fires for warmth, which, because of the smoke, made their whereabouts more visible. Europeans also attacked the Khoikhoi pastoralists, stealing stock, claiming grazing land and water, and murdering Khoikhoi people. The commandos were armed by the Dutch East India Company (VOC) (Adhikari, 2011). The genocidal attacks on the Khoisan are especially significant to this work because they constitute "an appreciable strain in the making of the [C]oloured people" (79) of South Africa (Marais, 1939/1968).

Both the Khoikhoi and San people responded to these occupiers by forming raiding parties attacking the European settlements. The San, in particular, were skilled at using guerilla tactics—killing the European settlers and their stock, destroying crops, and burning down farmsteads in an attempt to drive the *trekboers* (settlers) from their land. They were aided in their efforts by farm servants, many of whom had been captured by farmers and forced to work for them. Despite these efforts, the *trekboers* were at a distinct military advantage in the battles, having horses and using guns that could shoot twice the distance of a San arrow (Adhikari, 2011). In an attempt to calm the situation, the European authorities issued rules forbidding enslavement of the local Khoisan people. These rules were only halfheartedly issued and largely ignored, and therefore the battles continued. So many San and Khoikhoi were killed that the demand for labor surpassed the colonists' ability to capture San and Khoikhoi people, and Europeans began to "import" humans as slaves from other areas of the world.

Many of the first people enslaved in South Africa were brought from other places in Africa such as Angola and the Guinea Coast (Dooling, 2007). Eventually most people were brought from much farther away—especially from Indonesia, where the Dutch had similar designs of conquering, ruling, and exploiting the people and resources of Asia as well as southern Africa. Some of the people who were made to be slaves brought from East Asia by the Dutch were political prisoners. When Indonesians led protests against colonialism, the Dutch responded by branding them criminals and shipping them to South Africa to toil as slaves. Thousands of Malaysian people were kidnapped and brought in chains, especially to the Western Cape to work as slaves on wine and wheat estates (Dooling, 2007). The people who were enslaved often were literate and highly skilled craftspersons performing work ranging from construction to farming while others worked as domestic servants, wet nurses, artisans, fishermen, and gardeners (Beck, 2000).

Some individuals laboring as slaves were allowed to keep part of the money they earned from practicing their trades and were thereby able to purchase their freedom. Others were freed by the individuals who owned them. But these numbers were small, especially as slavery became entrenched in South Africa, and the laws held that children born of a slave mother retained their slave status. The large majority of the Coloured population was slaves (Beck, 2000).

Many of the people brought to the Cape from Asia were Muslims. As slaves they were allowed to practice Islam, but if they were found talking about their religion to others, they would be killed. While Coloured South Africans today hold many different religious beliefs, predominantly Islam and Christianity, Islam continues to play an especially important role in the community in the Western Cape (Jeppe, 2001).

Language is also an important feature of identity for Coloured South Africans. Afrikaans is the primary language for many, but not all, Coloured South Africans. It is a language with roots in Dutch spoken by European settlers from the Netherlands. In order to communicate, slaves and slaveholders began to adopt a version of the Dutch colonists' language intermixed with the languages of the Malaysians working as slaves as well as the languages of other peoples in southern Africa who were part of the broader community. Out of this mix, Afrikaans emerged. On a side note, during the heyday of apartheid, white Afrikaners claimed to be a white "tribe" based on their ancestry in Africa, their culture, and their language— Afrikaans. But in fact Afrikaans is an African language, since it has developed over the centuries in South Africa; what the Afrikaners neglected to acknowledge was that Coloured South Africans also shared this language (BBC, 1980).

The population of people laboring as slaves grew rapidly in the Cape from 337 in 1692 to 14,747 in 1793 and then at about a 2.5 percent annual increase during the eighteenth century. About 60,000 women and men were captured in other countries and brought to the Cape between 1652 and 1807, when the slave trade was ended. By the eighteenth century there were more people from outside southern Africa working as slaves than white European settlers living in the main farming areas. About two-thirds of the slave population lived on wine and wheat estates, while the other third resided in the city of Cape Town (Dooling, 2007; Ross, 1994; Worden, 1985). This community of urban and rural slaves formed the historical core of the Coloured community of South Africa.

The End of Slavery and the Creation of Apartheid

The Cape became occupied by the British near the end of the eighteenth century, but the British were not interested in investing troops or money to establish a stable colony there. Dutch farmers and merchants ran the economy and owned most of the land and the people who were slaves. The Cape, however, was officially governed by the British, and when the British government abolished the slave trade in 1808, slavery became illegal throughout most of the British Empire. There were a number of loopholes and exemptions, though, and it was not until December 1, 1838, that all of the individuals working as slaves in South Africa were officially freed. Most of these people left the estates where they had been held captive to make their way into the South African economy as freed persons. A few of them were very successful, but most former slaves continued to live in poverty and were subjected to discrimination and brutality (Dooling, 2007).

Early in the twentieth century, the British relinquished control of their colonial holdings in southern Africa to the local white population. These whites were also of European ancestry, but their ancestors had emigrated from the Netherlands centuries before and for years had fought the British unsuccessfully for control of South Africa. They called themselves Afrikaners. Although the British won the military victories and South Africa continued to nominally be a British dominion as the twentieth century began, Afrikaners had already gained political control. In 1910, Louis Botha, an Afrikaner, became the first prime minister in the Union of South Africa. Only eight years before his election he had unsuccessfully led Afrikaner troops against the British in a military attempt to take control from Britain.

After his election, Botha and his National Party passed the 1910 Act of Union, creating a single nation where only white South Africans were truly citizens. Over the next forty years, successive white governments passed laws further segregating and excluding all South Africans of color from economic, social, political, and physical arenas. The Land Act of 1913 limited people of colors' access to land in the nation as a whole, and the 1923 Natives (Urban Areas) Act established the principle that urban areas were for whites only. People of color were allowed into the cities only to work (Beck, 2000).

Official power was transferred from Britain to the Afrikaners in 1948. Based on the acts passed in the first half of the century, the Afrikaner government began to develop the policy of apartheid that lasted until 1994. Apartheid in Afrikaans means "separate" and "refers to the system of racial discrimination and white political domination adopted by the National Party while it was in power from 1948–1994" (Beck, 2000, p. 125). Apartheid was an elaborate system of racial segregation and discrimination. Under apartheid, Afrikaners developed an arbitrary system for racial classification of all people who were not white. The rights of people of color, or more often lack of rights, stemmed from their position within the system, "beginning with birth in a racially segregated hospital and ending with burial in a racially segregated cemetery. In between, South Africans lived, worked, and played out their lives at racially segregated offices, businesses, schools, colleges, beaches, restrooms, park benches, restaurants, theatres, and sports fields" (p. 125). Where one was allowed to live or even travel was determined by one's position within the segregated system. The right to vote or run for office was reserved for whites only. Eventually, even the choice of whom to marry or with whom to have sex were restricted by apartheid laws.

Apartheid, a political and judicial system constructed by the white South African government, was founded on the physical and social separation of people based on the racial classification system the whites had constructed (Salo, 2005). The white government, which represented only 13 percent of the total population, passed a series of acts to implement the apartheid system. The Population Registration Act of 1950 (and subsequent amendments) forced all South Africans into one of the four basic prescribed race categories:

> "A White person is one who in appearance is, or who is generally accepted as, a White person, but does not include a person who, although in appearance obviously a White person, is generally accepted as a Coloured person. A native is a person who is in fact or is generally accepted as a member of any aboriginal race or tribe of Africa. A Coloured person is a person who is not a White person nor a native." Later, a fourth category, Indian, was added, for people of South Asian descent; the label "native" was replaced by the labels "Bantu" and "Black." Racial classification was recorded in official identity documentation. From 1970, the "Black" category was further subdivided into ethnic or linguistic groups (such as Zulu and Xhosa). (Seekings, 2008, p. 3, quoting definitions of racial categories in government documents)

According to the government, the category "Coloured" included the descendants of relationships between white and black people and the descendants of Malaysian slaves brought from Southeast Asia. Descendants of Malaysian slaves were briefly categorized into their own "race" in 1951 but eventually collapsed into the "Coloured" category. In 1970 descendants of the indigenous Khoikhoi and San people who had resided in the Western Cape before the arrival of either white or black people and did not speak "Bantu" languages were added to the category of "Coloured" (Seekings, 2008).

In 1949 the Mixed Marriages Act and the Immorality Act prohibited people of color from marrying or having sexual relations with whites. Existing mixed marriages were nullified, and mixed couples who were caught having sex were imprisoned.

In other important government actions, the Group Areas Act of 1950 forced various categories of people of color to live in particular areas, and the Native Resettlement Act nullified existing property rights by zoning certain residential and trading zones as restricted to whites only and forcing millions of people of color from their homes and businesses (Beck, 2000). Members of the Coloured community, who had previously worked as slaves in urban areas and had continued after the abolition of slavery to live in closely knit communities in Cape Town for generations, were forcibly removed from their original neighborhoods and homes. The forced removals tore apart families and friends who had lived in close proximity for decades. People who had once relied on one another as friends and family members were forced to move far from where they had been raised. Not only were people ripped from their communities and made to live in new communities full of people they did not know, but the areas to which they were forced to move were barren and far removed from the city. These areas were without familiarity, decent housing, good land, and, most importantly, there were no jobs. White South Africans were then given their choice of land and properties that had once belonged to the people who had been forced to leave. Pass laws were enacted in these areas of displacement, and residents were required to carry and produce on demand identity documents. Much like "tags," "passes," and "free papers" required by law for black people traveling in the United States during the 1700s and 1800s during slavery, and like the recent requirements in several states in the United States that people appearing to be "foreign" present green cards on demand, only South Africans in possession of these documents were legally allowed to move outside of the confines of their designated neighborhood.

Whites were the only people allowed to live and work in the best areas. The Western Cape is a province on the west coast of South Africa. Its stunning beauty and rich farmland, the heart of the wine industry and centuries-old vineyards, made it one of the prime areas for white settlement. Cape Town is the major city in the Western Cape; in fact, it is the only really large city in the province. Cape Town and the leafy suburbs surrounding it were set aside for whites only.

In hospitals, patients were supposed to be handled by nurses of the "appropriate" racial group (although almost all doctors were white). Segregation was extended to other areas of social interaction: education (with separate schools and universities for each racial group), transport (separate railway carriages), and most municipal facilities, such as parks and beaches. Where complete segregation was not possible, partial segregation was implemented through separate entrances and counters (at railway stations and post offices, for example) (Seekings, 2008).

The apartheid system, however, could not entirely restrict people of color from going into "white areas," because their labor was needed to serve the needs of whites, so the system had to address the problem of providing that labor. In doing so, hierarchies within communities of color were created. All sorts of localized restrictions and rules were put in place. Legislation such as the Coloured Labour Preference Policy implemented in the 1950s, for example, gave preference to Coloured people as cheap sources of labor over black people in the textile and farming industries in the Western Cape (Salo, 2005). This policy allowed only some South Africans who were not white into some areas and created layers of inequities within the apartheid system.

Coloured people were permitted to live in very restricted areas within the Cape Town area. Black men, on the other hand, were even more excluded. They were allowed to live only in small hostels far away on the outskirts of the city from which they commuted, if their labor was needed there. Black women were also permitted into the city as live-in domestic workers. If their labor was not required, black people were not permitted into the Western Cape at all. Black South Africans were relegated to isolated barren areas far away from the white communities, cities, and good farmland. Only a few of the people designated by the apartheid system as Asian were allowed to migrate into the Western Cape, and most people whose ancestors had come from other Asian countries, particularly India, were confined to the provinces in eastern South Africa. Aslam Fataar (2007) writes:

> Whites were at the receiving end of state sponsored social privilege that secured them first-world living standards, while Black Africans were regarded as "temporary sojourners" who were not allowed to settle permanently in the city [of Cape Town]. The Coloured group, of which these teachers [in his study] were a part, was at the receiving end of a permanent settlement policy by the state in return for providing the city with cheap unskilled and semi-skilled labor. This ambivalent insider status marked the group's search for identity and place in South Africa. (p. 158)

Coloured people were "privileged" relative to black South Africans, because they were allowed closer access to the best areas to live and work in the Western Cape. Coloured people, however, were required to live only in designated areas within the areas designated as "whites only." When the apartheid government designated Cape Town and much of the surrounding countryside as an area where only whites were allowed, they had to first clear out the Coloured people who had lived there for hundreds of years.

Relocation in Apartheid South Africa

For centuries, first as slaves and then after the abolition of slavery as laborers, artisans, and fisherfolk, Coloured people had resided in neighborhoods within Cape Town, especially in the central areas such as Claremont, District Six, Kirstenbosch, and Simon's Town. The apartheid government removed people as part of their ethnic cleansing. Coloured people were forced to move to the sand dunes, far away from the city centers, designated as the "Cape Flats." In some cases their homes were bulldozed and apartments and new houses for whites were put up on the sites—for example, in District Six (Beyers, 2008). In other areas in the central city, the houses remained but were taken over by whites. Bo Kaap, which is in downtown Cape Town, was one area that was set aside for Muslims, most of whom were Coloured and whose families had lived there continuously since the 1600s, when they were brought into the country as slaves. The middle-class Coloured residents of Bo Kaap were able to retain their homes through the period of removals, and they remain there today, although gentrification by wealthy white people is now rapidly encroaching on the community.

In 1950 the Group Areas Act led to the forced removal of millions of people in South Africa. In the Western Cape, mostly Coloured people were evicted from mixed residential areas when they were declared "white" areas (Seekings, 2008). For example, the 1951 census reported that in a suburb of Cape Town called Claremont the population consisted of 19,811 whites, 18,278 Coloureds, and 507 black South Africans. All of the Coloured and black residents were forced to leave. People were collected from their homes like cattle. They were forced to gather their belongings and were loaded onto the back of trucks. Even today, older Capetonians are still able to describe in vivid detail these traumatic events that took place sixty years ago. Black South Africans had already been largely excluded several decades earlier, but the community was a nearly equal mix of white and Coloured people in the years immediately before apartheid. After the Group Areas Act was implemented, it was exclusively white, and it remains predominantly white today even though the act was repealed in 1991. Nearly a decade after the fall of the apartheid government, Wiesahl Taliep (2001) wrote, "Claremont today, with its many expensive homes and upmarket shopping malls, epitomizes white middle-class culture in Cape Town" (p. 65).

The forced removals were traumatic both economically and socially. Coloured residents were forced to leave in haste, even though housing on the Cape Flats was often still unavailable, and new arrivals had to make do with any temporary accommodation they could find. There were severe penalties for not leaving quickly. Most people were forced to leave with no compensation whatsoever. But the government offered to compensate some people who had been "disqualified" from the now whites-only area if they had legal documents proving they owned the property. If they did not leave within one year, however, they had to remit 25 percent of whatever excess they made on the sale of their house. After two years they were required to remit 50 percent. For those whom the act provided compensation for expropriated land, the amount was determined by the Department of Community Development, the same people who were implementing the relocations. "Disqualified persons" were often paid only a fraction of the actual worth of their property (Taliep, 2001). One man who was forced to relocate explained to a journalist at the time: "It makes me bitter that the home for which my father toiled in since 1901 should be taken from us. I have owned that house for 30 years. A man struggles for his children and when he can work no longer his children struggle . . . what happens to the family? For what have his children struggled?" (*Cape Argus,* 28 Oct. 1964, cited in Taliep, 2001).

For those lucky enough to find shelter in the areas to which they had been relocated, the conditions of life were difficult in the undeveloped area without amenities, even those as basic as indoor plumbing or running water (Taliep, 2001). Many were simply unable to find housing at all. By 1966 there were over 10,000 Coloured people on the waiting list for houses in Cape Town (*Cape Argus,* 24 June 1966, cited in Taliep, 2001). The housing shortage became critical as more areas were declared white and more Coloured families were evicted. By 1969 the shortage had increased to between 15,000 and 20,000 without housing in the Cape Peninsula (*Cape Argus,* 18 Nov. 1969, cited in Taliep, 2001).

Not only were homes lost, but the livelihoods of shopkeepers and traders were also destroyed when "disqualified persons" lost their trading licenses along with their right of occupation. Once they were relocated far away from the city, the lively small shops—the general-goods dealers, butcher shops, tailor shops, shoe repair and shoe shops—automatically lost their long-established clientele. Businesses failed and people were left with neither housing nor income (Taliep, 2001). The structural changes that destroyed communities, jobs, and homes along with the psychological trauma of these changes and the removals themselves created new neighborhoods with high levels of unemployment, crime, and alcohol and drug abuse.

Afrikaans

Throughout this history of slavery and apartheid, Coloured people worked for white employers, both English and Afrikaners. The Afrikaans language continued to develop and became common to Coloured employees and white employers (Cohen, 2007). Today, South Africa has eleven official languages. Afrikaans (13.3 percent of South Africans speak this as a first language) is the language of many whites whose ancestors came from the Netherlands. Other white South Africans have British roots and speak English as a first language (8.2 percent of all South Africans speak English as a first language). The dominant African languages are isiZulu (23.8 percent) and isiXhosa (17.6 percent), and there are a number of others that are the first language of many black South Africans, including Sepedi (9.4 percent), Sesotho (7.9 percent), Xitsonga (4.4 percent), siSwati (2.7 percent), Tshivenda (2.3 percent), and isiNdebele (1.6 percent).

Among Coloured South Africans, Afrikaans is the dominant language. About 80 percent of Coloured South Africans speak Afrikaans as their first language. In addition, Coloured people usually speak two versions of Afrikaans: the form spoken by whites and the form spoken by the Coloured community. The other 19 percent of Coloured South Africans speak English as a first language (Statistics South Africa, 2004). Many Coloured people also read and sometimes speak Arabic if it is the language of their religion, Islam.

A Question of Identity

Abebe Zegye (2002) writes, "[W]hen thinking of 'colouredness' in South Africa, the complexities of living the legacy of this category make it difficult to generalize about what it means to be 'coloured'" (p. 323). And while we have attempted to sketch just some of the historical roots of "colouredness," the question of who are Coloured people and what comprises this culture is a long debated issue. The term or category "Coloured" was created largely by external forces that first kidnapped and enslaved people in Asia and forced their migration to South Africa and then defined these peoples' borders by arbitrary definitions, adding people on the basis of skin color and ancestry. Some scholars argue that this ambiguity has meant that Coloured people have no identifiable culture. Ethnic studies scholars have defined ethnic groups as people who share a language, culture, and history, but Coloured South Africans are heterogeneous in all of these areas. They speak Afrikaans, English, or a mix of both. Some Coloured people whose ancestors were brought from Asia share a history of slavery, while others whose ancestors were Khoisan share a different history. Their culture varies from the highly urban experience of Coloured Capetonians in Salt River to the rural Coloured communities in the wine lands of Paarl and Worcester (Petrus & Isaacs-Martin, 2011).

Zegeye (2002) argues that Coloured South Africans have multiple identities based on regionalism, language, and ideology. In addition, he maintains that scholars have perceived Coloured people as a minority within the country that did not warrant research, and therefore the problem of unraveling all of the diverse strands within the community to determine the multiple identities has remained unsolved (Grunebaum & Robins, 2001). Others, however, have pointed out that, despite the ambiguity, many Coloured people perceive themselves and are perceived by others as a racial ethnic other (Hendricks, 2001). In addition, some scholars assert that a well-integrated and remarkably stable culture is at the heart of the Coloured community (Adhikari, 2006).

Mohamed Adhikari is one of those scholars who has grappled with this problem and shares the position of this latter group. He maintains that Coloured South Africans have a clear, consistent culture marked by three factors, all of which contributed to the marginality of the Coloured community and severely limited their options for social and political action: assimilationism, intermediate status in the racial hierarchy, and negative connotations of being racially mixed.

Assimilationism is the practice of becoming part of a dominant culture. It involves adopting the culture, values, and behaviors of those who are at the top of the social hierarchy. Adhikari argues that the Coloured community, especially those people who were able to obtain an education or to succeed financially, sought to become more like the ruling elite, white Afrikaners. The quest to assimilate was spurred by hopes of acceptance into the dominant society and therefore access to the education, houses, and eventually civil rights of the ruling whites. Coloured South Africans were not granted these rewards for attempts to assimilate, but their strategy was one of trying to blend in so that they might not be excluded.

Adhikari points to the intermediate status in the racial hierarchy as a second feature of Coloured identity. He observes the efficacy of the apartheid system, which created layers of inequality. Although Coloured people were given few rights within the system, they were not treated as harshly as black South Africans. The gap between the white population and everyone else was stunning. The gap between Coloured South Africans and black South Africans was smaller but visible. The "divide and conquer" strategy generated fears among Coloured South

Africans that they might lose their position of relative privilege and be relegated to the status of black South Africans.

The third significant factor of Coloured identity, according to Adhikari, is negative connotations of being racially mixed. By this he is referring to the stigma associated with Coloured people that defined them as less than both white and black South Africans because they were "not quite" either. Adhikari asserts that the dearth of scholarly work on Coloured history is one of the most telling indications of the marginality and invisibility of Coloured people in South Africa.

While Adhikari argues that these three factors are critical aspects of the identity and experience of Coloured South Africans, he also maintains that if scholars were to investigate Coloured history and culture, they would find a vibrant community. The real history and identity of Coloured South Africans would show that despite the struggle to assimilate, they were never able to lose themselves in the dominant culture by power of the white populations, nor the dominant cultures by numbers of black South Africans. This in-between intermediate status coupled with struggles with the tensions of slavery, colonialism, and apartheid molded Coloured people into an identifiable, coherent culture and community of their own.

Recent empirical studies have found evidence of some of Adhikari's ideas. Matthew Taylor and his colleagues (Taylor, Mwaba & Rule, 2011), for example, found that participants identified themselves as Coloured as a distinct category within South Africa that was neither white nor black. The criteria they used to describe their identity included speech (a particular way of speaking Afrikaans, English, and a mix of these), food (including various curries, bredies, and barbecued or *braaied* meats), dress (which included a general attention to the importance of appearance and clothing as well as more specific fashions), and neighborhood (named communities in the Cape Town area such as Manenberg). They also described some of the negative stereotypes and subsequent stigmatization they believe have become associated with Coloured identity, such as gangsterism, drug and alcohol abuse, and adolescent pregnancy. In addition, participants in the study explained their feeling of continuing marginalization and their belief that white people used to be in charge of South Africa, and now black people are, while Coloured people continue to be excluded (Taylor et al., 2011).

Eliminating Race and Racism in Revolutionary South Africa

In the mid-1990s, revolutionary forces under the direction of the African National Congress (ANC) toppled the apartheid regime and held democratic elections to begin a new era in South Africa. Nelson Mandela, the candidate of the ANC party, was elected the first president in 1994 and the long, difficult task of rebuilding a nation began. A new constitution was written, and new laws and social institutions were put into place to correct the wrongs of apartheid.

When political forces began to organize against apartheid, they worked for unity among all oppressed people and called for the elimination of the names that had been created or institutionalized by the apartheid government and had created cleavages among South Africans. In revolutionary South Africa, all oppressed groups called themselves "black." The term "Coloured" became a mark of the old system that the Coloured community, as well as those revolutionaries who had been previously identified as black by the apartheid government, wished to abolish.

In addition to this general need for unity, the lines between the different groups of people needed to be eliminated because the apartheid system had practiced a strategy of divide and conquer, writing elaborate rules that granted small privileges to some over others. For example, as we saw earlier in this chapter, Coloured people had been removed from the best places to live and work and had seen their houses ripped from them as they were forced out onto the sandy plains east of Cape Town. But during this same period, only a few black South Africans were even allowed into the Western Cape, and those who were granted work passes were allowed to live in only the worst conditions. Some of the Coloured community had gone along with this, perhaps in hopes of eventually assimilating into white society and being given full privileges and rights. At every turn, the apartheid government showed that it had no intention of granting anything near equality, but there were some small benefits.

Attempts to eliminate the term "Coloured" and the barriers between black South Africans and Coloured South Africans was a noble and essential part of the struggle. The identity of Coloured, however, persists. Coloured people continue to use the term to describe themselves and continue to search for and express their identity as distinct from the many ethnic communities within South Africa. The persistence of the use of the term "Coloured" as a way to describe oneself is perhaps one way of asserting a distinct identity.

In Between

The Coloured community today remains "in between," rarely as wealthy as many white South Africans but frequently better off than most black South Africans. While Cape Town is much more integrated than during the apartheid years, housing remains quite segregated, and Coloured residential areas are sandwiched in between the beautiful villas in the foothills, nearly all white, and the impoverished townships such as Khayelitsha, far from the city center, which are mostly populated by black South Africans. Many Coloured residential areas are concentrated on the plains situated between these two. The Coloured community is politically segregated as well. Uneasy with the ANC, which has been perceived by many Coloured South Africans as having the interests of only black South Africans, Coloured voters have sometimes gone so far as to support the old political parties of apartheid as well as new conservative parties. Many Coloured people see the ANC as a party of black elites. They argue that the ANC has gone too far in its quest to empower previously excluded people, especially those who found themselves at the very bottom of the racial hierarchies during apartheid. The government of South Africa today is democratically representative at least in terms of skin color, which means that black South Africans are in the leadership positions. Coloured South Africans are a minority and therefore do not wield as much power. Some Coloured South Africans complain that they were not white enough for the apartheid government and now they are not black enough to be fully acceptable to the current government (Zegeye, 2002) reinforcing a discourse of "in-betweeness."

Today many Coloured people still live in segregated neighborhoods on the outskirts of Cape Town. If they can find paid employment, weak public transportation systems and the long distances between Coloured neighborhoods and places of employment in the city center make it expensive and difficult to get work. The problem of poverty remains significant for a large proportion of Coloured people. Ironically, women historically sometimes fared better than men within the system of apartheid. Although Coloured women were subject to restrictions and oppression under patriarchy, at the same time they had an advantage over Coloured men in the labor market. When it came to working for wages, women were often the primary breadwinners (Salo, 2005) as a result of the historical importance of the textile industry to the economy of the Western Cape.

Coloured women continue to play a significant role in the labor market, although the gaps between themselves and women in other population groups are no longer as significant. In 2005, 77.9 percent of Coloured men were in the labor market and 66.3 percent of Coloured women were in the labor market. Although the gap between Coloured women and women in other population groups has shrunk, Coloured women today are still more likely to be in the labor market than are black women (64.1 percent), white women (62 percent), and Asian women (54.4 percent) (Botshabelo & Nakanyane, 2006).

In addition, under apartheid, women, at least those who were mothers, received preference over men for the allocation of housing and social grants. The apartheid government would not grant child welfare grants and public housing to families other than nuclear families. Children were most often in the care of their mothers, which meant women were more likely to apply for welfare as a family, while men would be perceived as single and without a family (Salo, 2005). These circumstances created an unusual situation for Coloured women and, to a lesser extent, black women living in the Western Cape.

Today, however, poverty remains a significant problem for the majority of South Africans, and gender hierarchies do not benefit women. In a large quantitative study of poverty using a wide range of variables, including access to housing, sanitation, electricity, clean water, household expenditures, employment status, and education in the Western Cape, Serumaga-Zake, Kotze, and Madsen (2005) found that large proportions of the population were living in difficult circumstances. The most vulnerable were urban households headed by black women, black men, Coloured women, and Coloured men in that order.

The Coloured community of South Africa has faced many difficulties in its long history, beginning with slavery and colonialism and moving through the apartheid era. Today apartheid is legally gone, but Coloured people still often live in segregated and impoverished neighborhoods. In the early 1980s another challenge emerged and continues to cause immense problems: HIV. Today the virus affects and infects large sections of the South African population.

A new nationwide study of HIV prevalence is currently under way by the Human Sciences Research Council in South Africa. The last nationally representative study was conducted in 2008 (Shisana et al., 2009). The latest figures report that the Western Cape had the lowest HIV prevalence in the country. Women (13.6 percent) had a higher prevalence of HIV than men (7.9 percent), with black women ages 20 to 34 having the highest prevalence overall. The Coloured population group had the next highest prevalence (1.7 percent) of HIV in the country after blacks (13.6 percent). This data on the racial distribution of HIV prevalence has not been analyzed by gender, so it is not clear what the picture looks like for Coloured women compared to Coloured men or other women. However, given that the burden of HIV is overwhelmingly borne by women (these data are consistent throughout the surveys in 2002, 2005, and 2008), one can assume that this will not be any different for Coloured women. Coloured and black South Africans are among those hard hit by HIV, and therefore they are the focus of this research. Our research for this book tells the stories of a support group of Coloured HIV-positive women living in Cape Town, South Africa.

The stories reflect the social context of the women's lives. The legacy of slavery and apartheid and the remaining racial-ethnic and social-class inequalities shape the experience women have as they cope with the challenges of living with HIV. Although their access to support groups and ARVs has been greatly improved by the country's progress in supporting people living with HIV, poverty, racism, and sexism remain barriers to securing the adequate wages, income, housing, and transportation women need to survive. At every turn these structural failures in the labor market, the social welfare system, and the general broad array of social institutions shape the problems women face and the options that are available to cope with or solve those problems.

3 A Support Group for HIV-Positive Women in Cape Town

THE FIRST CASES of HIV were identified in South Africa in the early 1980s. The numbers affected by the epidemic grew fairly slowly in the 1980s and early 1990s but exploded in the late 1990s and the first decade of the twenty-first century. At first the government was unprepared to deal with the problem. Then in 1998, AZT (azidothymidine), an antiretroviral drug especially useful for inhibiting mother-to-child infection, became available to those who could afford to buy the medicine. Initial distribution of AZT faltered when the South African government decided it was too expensive, and the health minister said the state's primary focus would be on prevention rather than treatment. The government continued to drag its feet in making the drug available, claiming it was concerned about the efficacy and potential dangers of antiretroviral medicines. As recently as 2005, government officials continued to issue controversial and scientifically unsubstantiated justifications for not providing ARVs to HIV-positive people in South Africa. Some HIV activists in South Africa, as well as people in government, were vocal about their skepticism regarding the efficacy and safety of ARVs. A few went so far as to question whether the new drugs were yet another deadly experiment the West was conducting in Africa. This view, however, is unquestionably a minority one, although it has been articulated by some of the most powerful people in the country. Former South African health minister Manto Tshabalala-Msimang, for example, endorsed foods such as garlic, beetroot, and lemon juice as valid alternatives to ARVs for the treatment of HIV. She argued her position in national discussions and before the world in a speech at the International AIDS Conference in Toronto in 2006 (Lewis, 2006), but her speeches were immediately condemned around the globe, most vehemently from within South Africa. More recently, skepticism about ARVs has waned as people in countries who previously did not have access to them are finally able to use at least some of the medicines and see the real and positive effects of the drugs.

The Treatment Action Campaign (TAC), the most vocal activist organization in South Africa for the rights and treatment of people living with HIV and for the prevention of new infections, makes a human rights argument asserting that it is the right of people living with HIV to receive access to ARVs in a timely manner (Seidel, 1993). The TAC (2007) posits that it is a breach of the South African Constitution and of human rights if all persons living with HIV do not have access to ARVs.

A broad, sustained political battle was waged by organizations aligned with the TAC to challenge the government, and through their efforts ARV medicines began to be distributed throughout the nation in 2003. Zackie Achmat, a leader in the TAC and a Nobel Peace Prize nominee who is HIV positive, led the campaign by refusing to use ARVs until they were available in all provinces in South Africa. He was joined by five thousand scientists who signed the Durban Declaration in 2000 demanding that the government stop ignoring the science and move to provide South Africans with the highly effective ARVs. Activists marched in the streets of South Africa and followed government officials to national and international gatherings to expose the government's unwillingness to support ARVs, pointing out the huge numbers of people who were dying as a result of the government's inaction. As the battle between antiretroviral advocates and the national government continued, several provinces began their own rollout programs to distribute ARVs. In 1999 the Western Cape was the first province to take this action.

ARV medications and rollout programs for the treatment of HIV infections have become somewhat more available recently, especially in certain nations in the Global South that previously had little access to the drugs. Lekas and her colleagues (2006, p. 1165), in the United States, refer to the year 2000 and beyond as the "HAART era" (HAART meaning "highly active antiretroviral treatment"), and the first decade of the twenty-first century was significant in the expansion of the treatment and distribution of ARVs in the treatment of HIV worldwide. In South Africa the Antiretroviral Treatment Protocol (Provincial Administration Western Cape, 2004) for the Western Cape was released in 2004. These improvements in accessibility and in the drugs themselves are welcome, but the issue of ARV treatment remains a complex and often controversial one.

Convincing arguments have been made for and against the implementation of ARV rollout plans, especially in South Africa, where HIV activists have been vocal in both the national and international arenas on the issue. The activist discourse not only promotes the idea that people have rights to access knowledge and treatment generated by scientific research. It also asserts that people of African countries, and other countries where ARV drugs are being tested on humans, have rights and must be granted the benefits of the medications, specifically because through their participation in drug testing it is they who have furthered the development of the treatments (Seidel, 1993). The activist discourse has not been uniformly accepted—for example, in highly controversial comments made by former President Mbeki—and public debate remains as to the value of ARVs. The activist discourse, however, is central to public debates regarding HIV and is undoubtedly a dominant position articulated in South Africa. In addition, the most recent discussions in the scientific community point to ARVs as a way to contain HIV and, eventually, to eliminate it from human populations. ARVs lower the viral load of people who are HIV positive to very small amounts, which makes it much less likely for people to infect others, even if they participate in unprotected sex (Sample, 2010).

In addition, the TAC endorsed the International AIDS Vaccine Initiative (IAVI), which involved human trials conducted in several places in the world, including South Africa. But vaccines have a large price tag. Pharmaceutical companies usually do not spend much money on developing drugs and vaccines that target the poorest nations in the world; for example, little work is being done to develop drugs to eliminate malaria. HIV, however, is one disease that has been a priority for both stockholders of pharmaceutical companies and health-care needs in the Global South. Pharmaceutical companies have invested significant funds to develop HIV treatments and vaccines, but they also expect to reap the financial benefits of this market. People of poor nations, however, have also contributed significantly: first when they endure the human drug trials in the research to develop the drugs, and later when they become consumers of the products. They hope to benefit by making sure the distribution of the treatments extends to everyone who needs them, including people without financial means to cover the costs. The tension between the interests of stockholders in pharmaceutical companies and people of poor nations that have high rates of HIV remains, and despite some positive change the ARV struggle continues (Smitt et al., 2006; Swartz & Kagee, 2006).

Most people in the Global South still do not have access to ARVs. The costs are high, and even when monies are available, the drugs are difficult and inconvenient to distribute and use. Those who are able to surmount all of these barriers face problems caused by the drugs themselves. Many of those who need ARVs are unsure and fearful about what the pills are doing to their bodies (Pound et al., 2005). Side effects from ARVs, such as severe dizziness and nausea, can last up to several months. In addition to the pain and suffering endured, these kinds of side effects can be debilitating and may prevent people from carrying out essential tasks in their lives. For example, it may prevent women from taking care of their young children. To make matters worse, government policies do not always work to support people living with HIV in the most efficient manner. In South Africa, for example, some people are forced to choose between social disability grants and ARVs.

The country's Department of Social Development (2006) provides that South Africans who cannot work because of a disability, including disabilities due to HIV, are eligible for social disability grants. Considering the increasing cost of living in South Africa, especially in Cape Town, these grants are not enough to live on. Nevertheless, many people living with HIV have come to depend on them as at least a partial form of subsistence. The problem with the grants is that as a person living with HIV becomes healthier as a result of ARV therapy, they become ineligible for the disability grant, thus creating a terrible choice (Hardy & Richter, 2006). On one hand, a doctor may tell a person who has become ill from the virus that their viral load, and most importantly their CD4 count, is at the point at which there is a need for ARV therapy. On the other hand, if a person has come to rely on a social disability grant to support their family, they actually run the "risk" of improving their health to the point that the Department of Social Development deems the grant unnecessary (Hardy & Richter, 2006). This causes further problems for women in particular, because women, as we later describe in chapter 7, are responsible for caring for and supporting the people in their household. Many women may believe there is really no choice to be made between their own health and the daily needs of their children and other people whom they are supporting. Some women may choose to reject the ARV treatment, resulting in further deterioration of their physical as well as emotional health. The responsibilities of women for care work lead them to face an ironic and tragic dilemma between providing for their families and taking care of their own personal health.

Despite this history of controversy and the continued debates and dilemmas surrounding ARV policy, today South Africa has the largest antiretroviral therapy program in the world (Avert, 2010b). ARVs are distributed at thousands of community sites, including military centers and prisons. In addition, more than 14,000 health-care workers have been trained to administer the program (Benton, 2007). The program, however, is still falling short of the needs of the people. The South African Ministry of Health's goal was to distribute ARVs to 80 percent of those in need of medicines by 2009, but only 50 percent of people in need were in programs by that date. And although in 2011 it was announced that there had been an increase in the numbers of people accessing ARVs from 923,000 in 2010 to 1.4 million in 2011 (Avert, 2012), South Africa remains the country with the highest number of people living with HIV. While the government now supports the use of ARVs, efforts to do so are constrained by two important factors: (1) they lack money; and (2) they lack sufficient numbers of health-care workers to run the programs that require testing for HIV, providing counseling, distributing the drugs, and providing ongoing medical and emotional support (Govender, 2009).

One aspect of the ARV programs in South Africa that has developed in response to some of these needs, especially the need for emotional support, is the establishment of networks of support groups with links to the local community (Mundell, 2006). The need for support groups to help people living with HIV maintain the regimen of physical, social, and psychological care for themselves while facing myriad other difficulties was identified early on in the pandemic (Mail & Matheny, 1989). Support groups have become a ubiquitous feature of communities addressing HIV all over the world (Knox, 1989; Liamputtong, Hariavorn & Kiatying-Angsulee, 2009; Mundell, 2006; Rivero-Mendez, Dawson-Rose & Solis-Baez, 2010).

Support Groups

People living with HIV must contend with arduous problems, including discrimination, exclusion, and even abuse. Support groups are currently the main intervention strategy to address emotional consequences of these problems (Beckett & Rutan, 1990; Kalichman, Sikkema & Somlai, 1996; Martin, Riopelle, Steckart, Geshke & Lin, 2001; Mundell et al., 2011; Nokes, Chew & Altman, 2003).

Support groups come in many sizes and structures and meet in a range of formats (Foster, Stevens & Hall, 1994). All are designed, however, to provide people with a safe environment to talk about the virus, share experiences, listen to the stories of other individuals living with HIV, and access information (Brashers, Haas, Klingle & Neidig, 2000; Summers et al., 2000). Peer support is achieved through the sharing of experience with others who face similar difficult issues. Being with people with similar problems alleviates the feelings of isolation and loneliness that can accompany an illness that carries with it such a negative stigma (Adamsen, 2002). Support groups can help people to confront the reality of the illness, including the stigma, without becoming completely overwhelmed and discouraged (Chung & Magraw, 1992). Support groups may work toward a range of goals, including learning to trust oneself and others; recognizing the commonality of needs and problems; increasing self-acceptance, self-confidence, and self-respect; finding alternative ways to deal with conflict; increasing self-direction, authority, and responsibility toward oneself; becoming aware of one's choices; making specific plans for change; learning more effective social skills; becoming more sensitive to the needs and feeling of others; learning to confront others with care, concern, honesty, and directness; and clarifying one's values and deciding whether and how to modify them (Corey, 2000; Gillett & Parr, 2010; Mundell, 2006; Liamputtong et al., 2009; Visser & Mundell, 2008). Support groups also provide a forum for teaching and learning about health and positive living, because HIV is a long-term illness that is relieved by staying as healthy as possible.

Undoubtedly, these lofty goals are rarely all met, but even so, researchers have found that support groups do indeed play a positive role in their members' lives. Support groups for people living with HIV are especially good at helping participants cope with some of the problems that are specifically associated with the virus. For example, unlike most other serious illnesses, people who are HIV positive often find they lose support from their families when they disclose their status. Others who might find support are too afraid to disclose their status to those who are close to them, because they fear rejection and, therefore, are not able to get the support they require from such people. Thus, for some the support group becomes a new family and a circle of care (Mundell, 2006; Mundell et al., 2011; Visser & Mundell, 2008; Yalom, 1995).

When asked how they believe their participation has affected them, members of HIV support groups report that the most important benefits of the group are being able to share feelings, finding relief from being alone, discovering opportunities to obtain information on treatments and approaches to care, and being able to have their questions answered (Mundell, 2006). Other research has found that participation in HIV support groups is directly associated with increased feelings of hope (Hays, Chauncey & Tobey, 1990). In addition, the support increases long-term coping skills, decreases feelings of emotional stress, and increases social contact (Hedge & Glover, 1990). Furthermore, support groups enhance the quality of life of their members and may help people to reduce risky behavior (Martin et al., 2001; Nuñes, Raymond, Nicholas, Leuner & Webster, 1995).

Beyond these individual benefits for people living with HIV, support groups are also central factors in what medical anthropologists call therapeutic citizenship (Biehl, 2007; Nguyen, 2005; Robins, 2006). Claims to citizenship and belonging begin within the support group when members are empowered and can work collaboratively to make claims for rights to universal access to treatment as well as other health and social needs (Rhine, 2009). All of these forms of support for people seeking to cope with HIV, as well as those who are working as political activists to alter the social context, are essential.

HIV-Positive Women in a Support Group in Cape Town

The stories in this book come from a qualitative field study of a community voluntary support group on the outskirts of Cape Town, South Africa. Importantly, this area is one of the spaces created as a result of apartheid group-area policies and is a location to which Coloured people were forcibly removed. Fifteen in-depth interviews were conducted with women who were participating in the community support group. Additional data were gathered in the form of field notes through participant observation methods during support group meetings over a period of fifteen months. The support group is the only one of its kind in a neighborhood that is home to thousands of people. The community has a low income level, and people reside in small homes and apartments (public/council housing) as well as shacks made of corrugated metal and wood. In addition, many people live on the street or in informal shelters. The HIV support group is open to men and women who test positive at any of the several clinics and day hospitals in the area. We volunteered at the group, meeting with the members on a weekly basis; helping with projects such as preparing lunch and food parcels; and providing workshops on HIV risks, prevention, and care.

Poor Coloured women represent a significant proportion of people living with HIV in South Africa; therefore, this study chose to specifically focus on the experiences of this group of women. This is an especially important population because, while their numbers are substantial, their voices have not often been heard in social science research and in HIV research in particular. The women's participation in the support group indicates that they are actively concerned about HIV in their community and might, therefore, be more willing or interested than others in talking about their lives. Because the women had participated in many discussions in the support group, they had already given much thought to the issues we were addressing in our research. Their membership in the support group also made the women more accessible to our research. We were able to become participant observers in the group, and the women had a chance to get to know us well enough to establish positive relationships, and in some cases friendships, before we began conducting interviews.

The women we interviewed were of varying ages and backgrounds and were eligible to participate if they were a part of the support group and were comfortable with conducting the interviews in English. The interviews were conducted in English because this is our first language and only one of us speaks Afrikaans as a second language. The first language of most of the women interviewed is Afrikaans, the language we described in chapter 2, but all of the women also spoke English, so it was the language we all had in common.

The women ranged in age from 34 to 50 years. They had a variety of occupations, including factory work, domestic work, and security guard work. Some of the women were seeking work but were unemployed at the time of the interviews for various reasons, including disability due to their HIV status. All of the women were mothers, and their children ranged in age from newborn babies to adults. Eight of the women had men partners, including ex-husbands with whom they had reconciled; five of the women were married; and two of the women were single.

The majority of the members had originally been referred to the support group when they requested services regarding their HIV-positive status from their clinic or day hospital. Local medical facilities often recommend this particular support group to community members as the only option for those who cannot afford transportation to other parts of Cape Town in order to attend other support groups. The goal of this particular group is to offer services to HIV-positive community members for a limited amount of time with the goal of "graduating" members after approximately eight weeks in the group (although it is not uncommon for members to request longer membership). The group offers weekly support group meetings run by facilitators and volunteers, including members cum volunteers, and modest food parcels that are distributed on a monthly basis to people who qualify for them.

Asking Questions about Living with HIV

Our interviews with women in the support group dealt with issues of gender and the psychological and social problems that are encountered by women living with HIV. The interviews were organized into four broad sections: (1) background information; (2) issues related to stigma; (3) effects of emotional and psychological issues on the women's well-being; and (4) violence. We also had detailed follow-up questions prepared for use as needed.

In July 2006 a personal contact invited us to a community meeting in the area of Cape Town where the research eventually took place. This initial meeting included a number of local HIV, tuberculosis (TB), and poverty activists. These particular meetings take place monthly in a community center in a neighborhood close to the one where the support group is located. Attending this meeting led to an abundance of offers, including leads for interviewees and invitations from several local women's empowerment organizations as well as invitations for greatly needed volunteers at a Cape Town TB hospital. The meeting also led to an introduction to the head of the support group of which we were eventually to become a part.

After a short interview about the research intentions and permission from the group members, the head facilitator of the group invited us to become volunteers at the support group. We began attending weekly meetings and various other events, including volunteering in a soup kitchen run by the group. At each meeting an announcement was made that we were looking for women who would like to share their stories in a confidential discussion. Over the months, women began to approach us after the support group meetings and arrangements were made for interviews.

As the interviews began to be scheduled and conducted, we used the method of snowball sampling, which "identifies cases of interest from people who know people who know what cases are information rich" (Miles & Huberman, 1994, p. 28). This method is very often helpful when research topics are highly sensitive or stigmatized, as in the case of studying HIV. Women who participated in an interview were asked to suggest other individuals they thought might be interested in participating, and if the interview was a positive experience, they were also asked to pass the word on to other women who may be feeling hesitant about participating.

Before each interview we talked with the woman about the purpose of the interview and the general topics we would be addressing. Each woman was asked to sign an informed consent form that included a thorough description of the study and the rights of the participant. This form was also discussed verbally before the signing. We talked with each woman about the idea that interviews were a way for women's voices to be heard and a way for important and helpful ideas to be taken into account in the future treatment of women living with HIV. In addition, after a discussion with one of the facilitators, it was agreed that the interviews could be a way for women to confidentially make suggestions about the improvement of the support group. The interviewees were made aware of this before and after each interview, and most participants took advantage of the opportunity to comment. The suggestions made were reported back to the facilitator with careful consideration for confidentiality and were subsequently incorporated into the support group's practices. Group members returned to confirm their approval of several changes that were implemented as a result of their confidential suggestions.

Ethical Considerations

Given that the topics of our investigation were of a sensitive nature, great care was taken to ensure the women interviewed were unharmed physically or emotionally. Because women living with HIV are considered a vulnerable population by international ethics committees, extra care was taken in terms of the ethical considerations in our research. The anonymity and confidentiality of participants were protected at every stage. Interviews were conducted only with people who were over the age of 18, South African citizens, and mentally competent. Since the subject of HIV and the issues surrounding it can be stressful, we were especially careful to terminate any interview in which the participant became too emotional or upset. There were several instances when an interviewee began to cry; when this happened, the recorder was turned off and we took a break. During these breaks we explained that the interview should not cause pain, that stopping early was not a problem, and that in fact it was their right to stop whenever they wished. In each instance, however, the women insisted that the interview should continue, citing it as one of the only times they had the opportunity to share personal information about their lives and HIV with the guarantee of complete anonymity. In fact, several women told us that a weight had been lifted and that the interview had given them a perspective on their lives that they had not considered before. The women also emphasized their need to communicate their experiences in order to ultimately improve the treatment of others who had been more recently diagnosed and were now facing what they had already gone through.

Our Role in the Research

Qualitative feminist research accords attention to a critical examination of the role of the researcher in the data collection process and throughout the research endeavor. In this section we highlight our positioning as being responsible for initiating and carrying out this study. For qualitative feminist researchers, this process is called reflexivity, and it is referred to as a "process" because it is ongoing throughout every step of a research project. Before data collection even begins, researchers affect their research—for example, by deciding on what the research questions are, how the data will be collected, and how the research will be framed. The data collection process itself is an interaction between two people. Like any conversation, what is said in an interview depends on who is in the room, what they think and feel about one another, and how they behave. If we want to produce meaningful research, we must be sure that we acknowledge the fact that interviews are subjective—they are shaped by the humans who are engaging in a social interaction. Once data have been collected and transcribed, researchers have an effect on the analysis, because they are able to shape research by extracting certain sections of the text to highlight an area of interest. As much as they may try to be objective in their collection and reporting of the data, researchers inevitably have an effect on the process and the product. Part of understanding the data collected in qualitative interviews is highlighting dominant discourses as they operate in society. In the next chapter we describe some of the dominant discourses that have emerged around the topic of HIV among policy makers, professionals, and activists. But it is also important to acknowledge that the researcher-participant interaction during this research elicited particular kinds of discourse as well. In other words, research is not carried out in a vacuum—the participants and researchers react to each other in many and changing ways. In fact, Naples (2003) advises that both participants and researchers play a major role in "shaping what we come to know about their lives and the communities in which they live and work" (p. 37).

A crucial factor affecting the reactions of the researchers and participants and the interactions between them is power. As feminist researchers, we are particularly concerned with being aware of and attempting to minimize any negative consequences of power imbalances in an interview between researchers and participants (Mies, 1983). One must be especially cognizant of the impact of power differentials in three areas: (1) power imbalances due to demographic differences; (2) power imbalances due to the nature of the methodologies regarding whether or not the research is a relatively equal exchange or exploitative; and (3) power exertion in reporting of the data (Wolf, 1996).

In most cases it is not possible to control for the effects of demographic differences between researchers and research participants. The participants we spoke to and with whom we worked in the support group live in impoverished conditions. Most of the women in the support group live in small homes without plumbing and electricity, and they speak openly about their struggles to find food (even a loaf of bread) each day. We found this to be the most painful part of working with the support group both for us and for the members of the group; we researchers are privileged in comparison to the other women in the group because of our education and subsequent access to employment and decent housing, food, and transport. It is also true that researchers often benefit more from the research they conduct than do the participants of the research who provide the valuable information (Scanlon, 1993). To some extent this imbalance is impossible to rectify. In almost all cases, researchers are in relative positions of power compared to research participants. And how could someone ever really be adequately compensated for the sharing of such sensitive information about some of the most private and painful aspects of their lives? Feminist methodology would contend that the best approach is to take steps to minimize this gap in power while still being aware that some injustice remains. We and the participants were aware of this socioeconomic imbalance, and the step we took to alleviate the power imbalance and provide some element of compensation was to engage in reciprocal research practices by continuing to volunteer at the support group beyond the time it took to collect the interviews and by offering our time and some of our resources in an attempt to diminish the power gap. For example, we regularly brought pots of food to support group meetings and dropped off bags of donated clothes and shoes to several women's homes. We also made ourselves available to group members in need of transport and regularly drove members to and from group meetings and on errands to social services offices and the homes of family members. We made announcements during meetings inviting members to call upon us to help search for employment opportunities and creating resumes. Presentations were made to the group regarding several medical care aspects of living with HIV. Members also used our voices as a confidential conduit between themselves and the group facilitators, enabling members to make suggestions about how to improve the support group's services.

Another important aspect of feminist methodology, besides offering participants something in return for their interviews, is the idea of making research findings accessible, especially in order to facilitate positive social change. As a reflection of our commitment to feminist methodology, we have presented the findings of the research to the facilitators of the support group organization so that they might be useful for creating positive social change (Reinharz, 1992). The latter activity was especially important because when women's suggestions were passed on to facilitators, one facilitator was able to use the women's ideas we had documented in our research in conjunction with information gained in her classes at a larger training organization called ATTIC (AIDS Training Information and Counseling Centre). ATTIC is the official training center established by the South Africa National Department of Health for people working in the field of HIV, an important source of policy for the women in the support group. In this way the group was able to implement new ideas and services in response to the members' needs and suggestions. One of the facilitators has also shared the findings of our research with other support groups and activists in the area. The publication of this book is another way for the voices of the women we interviewed to be heard around the world.

While this collaboration among the women in the support group, the facilitators, and us was successful, differences between the researchers and the women interviewed remained significant. Determining what those differences were and how they were significant, however, is no easy task. It is important to attempt to be aware of all forms of difference, but this process of reflexivity is not a simple or clear part of the research process. The problem lies in what Naples (2003) describes as the "Insider/Outsider Debate." Often there are no distinct lines drawn between researchers and participants, and even then the lines are ever changing. In our study when we entered the support group, we initially were perceived as outsiders. The facilitators, volunteers, and members knew us based only on our status as researchers from the University of Cape Town. In the beginning, therefore, these outsider markers had facilitators on their toes emphasizing issues such as their "transparency as an NGO" and the need for members to be on time and attend all meetings as if we were investigating the organization from a funder's point of view. The group members themselves were quiet but friendly in a formal way during this time. Slowly it became clear that we were attending the meetings not only as a way to conduct research, but also to get to know people in a community that is in close proximity and in some ways similar demographically to our own; to offer services as volunteers; and, most importantly, to act as a conduit between members, facilitators, and, ultimately, policy makers. Our status as outsiders evolved as we collected the interviews and as members of the group began to understand our goals and realized that some of our family members were also members of the same community in which the support group operated and of similar communities close by.

The most obvious "Insider/Outsider" issue was, of course, HIV status. We noted that the facilitators were quick to emphasize that they were HIV negative and that they frequently pointed out to group members this difference between themselves. In some cases there was an air of judgment as if to say, "I am a facilitator because I made good decisions regarding HIV infection, and now I am here to help all you poor people living with HIV." In fact, at one meeting one of the facilitators said, "We all have choices and you all made a bad choice, but your bed is made and now you must lie in it" (field notes, April 2007).

This distinction between positive and negative HIV status that was made by several of the facilitators seemed to have had an impact on the members in that they noticeably deferred to people who visited the group with a perceived negative status; we were people who were assumed to be HIV negative. Because of this situation, we made a point of regularly emphasizing the fact that becoming infected with HIV is not the result of a "bad choice" and that *anyone* is vulnerable to the virus at any time in their lives regardless of their current status. For this, we believe an insider status of sorts was granted to us by some members. It seemed as though participants felt as comfortable as could be possible discussing events leading up to their positive HIV tests, in that we too are women who are vulnerable to this same virus and were not interested in placing blame or labeling group members as people who made "wrong choices."

Understanding and Analyzing the Data

A theoretical framework is the perspective or approach that a researcher takes in order to understand a particular phenomenon or social problem. In chapter 1 we noted that in this book we have taken a critical postcolonial feminist approach to exploring the problem of HIV. From this perspective, a fundamental goal of our research was to hear the voices of women who have been marginalized not only by gender but also by race ethnicity, social class, and their position in the global world of North-South inequality.

The feminist approach used in this study is situated within a social constructionist paradigm. Social constructionism has been defined as "the research approach that seeks to analyze how signs and images have powers to create particular representations of people and objects—representations that underlie our experience of these people and objects" (Terre Blanche, Durrheim & Painter, 2006, p. 278). What this means is that when we interact with one another, we are constructing what we come to understand as reality. Social reality is not something that exists outside of us; rather, it is something that we are actively involved in creating as we interact with one another. To illustrate this we can look at the example of race. Race is commonly thought of as something "real," which is visible and biological. We think of race as something in our social experience that is a natural given rooted in our physical bodies. Anne Fausto-Sterling (2012) explains, however, that "there is wide biological variation in human traits, but because groups of traits don't link and vary together, this variation can't be used to set up clear racial categories." Race, in fact, is not something that is biological or something that we can determine by examining human genes—race does not exist as a real, scientifically measurable factor among humans. Race is not a natural aspect of being human, and the human species is not divided into real categories by race. Nevertheless, race is a powerful issue in our lives. It comes to be real because of the social meaning we attach to categories that have been arbitrarily constructed by those in power who wish to create human hierarchies in order to divide and exploit for various reasons. It is maintained and reproduced as people within a racist system continue to make it real in their everyday interactions. In the context of South Africa, this is illustrated in the racial classification system constructed by the apartheid regime. The racial categories were arbitrary, as we can see from evidence presented in chapter 2 about Coloured people. The apartheid government lumped lots of different population groups into a category they named Coloured. And this was done with the explicit purpose of controlling resources, controlling labor, and maintaining a social system where those in power remained in power. People living within the apartheid system experienced race as something real, and they perpetuated the categories and inequalities in their thinking and behavior as they interacted with each other. Today, although apartheid is no longer part of the legal system, the concept of race continues to be part of the way people think about themselves and others, the ways they interact with each other, and the ways they talk about their ideas and behaviors.

Social constructionists focus on how we create and maintain social constructs such as race. They assert that this process of constructing social relationships is especially related to the ways we use language (Flick, 2006). In the case of race, for example, it is important to listen to the words that are used and the meaning of the images and language people use in their description of race. In fact, the term "race" itself helps to perpetuate the idea that race is a real biological category. Today in South Africa scholars and governmental documents use the term "population group" rather than "race" to create a different way of thinking about and experience differences that do not reify race. (In contrast, in the United States the government uses the term "race" to categorize people and has created an elaborate system in government documents, such as the census, that help to perpetuate the idea that race is a real biological category.) In our research we focus on the social construction of HIV in the discourse of people who are living with HIV.

Discourse

Discourse can be defined as "broad patterns of talk—systems of statements—that are taken up in particular speeches and conversations, not the speeches or conversations themselves" (Terre Blanche, Durrheim & Painter, 1999, p. 156). Social constructionists are concerned with looking at these broad patterns of talk to see how they are constructed. How does the way we talk about social issues—our discourse—shape or even determine the ways we think about those issues, and how does our discourse make some social actions possible and others unthinkable? (Butler, 2006). Critical discourse analysis also emphasizes the issue of power. Not only are we looking at how discourse shapes ourselves and our world, but we are also examining why it is organized as it is, and specifically what social relationships are revealed in the discourses surrounding HIV. What relationships of power are embedded within discourse of HIV and issues that are related to it? Foucault (1980) is a central figure in the development of our ideas about discourse and its political meaning. He argues that power and relationships between the powerful and the subordinate are disclosed in discourse. He maintains that discourses are "system[s] of statements which cohere around common meanings and values . . . [that] are a product of social factors, of powers and practices, rather than an individual's set of ideas" (Hollway, 1983, p. 231). In the case of HIV, discourse abounds in medical settings, the media, government, and education. The dominant discourses surrounding HIV have an impact not only on what the world believes about HIV but also on how the research on the virus proceeds. Most importantly, dominant discourses have direct and indirect effects on the very people living with the virus.

According to Wodak and Meyer (2001), dominant or hegemonic discourses can be thought of as the general knowledge a population has about one idea or another. This knowledge in the form of discourse is not, however, a benign set of ideas for the education of the public. Foucault (1978) explains that knowledge does not make the "knower" smarter or more powerful. Instead, knowledge can be used as a tool by which powerful people exert power and control over less powerful people by telling them what to know and why. Knowledge can be a way of seeing and understanding the world that powerful people "feed" to the less powerful in order to keep them from demanding justice or from even seeing injustice. Discourse is a vehicle by which knowledge can be disseminated.

These dominant discourses with which power is wielded are the ideas that tend to support and reproduce the status quo, thereby helping to maintain existing power relations. Dominant discourses, however, do not appear to be dominating; rather, they "appear 'natural,' denying their own partiality and gaining their authority by appealing to common sense" (Gavey, 1989, p. 464). Dominant discourse is "hidden" from the casual observer and can appear inevitable, making other ideas unthinkable. But listening carefully to the voices of marginalized women who are not part of the dominant discourse and analyzing their ideas through discourse analysis allows one to peek beneath the discourse about issues such as HIV in order to learn about alternative experiences and opinions.

Foucault (1980) reminds us that dominant discourse is not the only form of discourse. Power is contested and resistance discourses are an aspect of struggles over power. Disclosing and understanding dominant discourse, its variations, and resistance discourse, as well, are therefore essential to understanding the experience and behaviors of people, powerful and subordinate, who are part of those discourses. In order to challenge relationships of power, we must first expose which mechanisms are maintaining them and which are challenging them.

Five discourses emerged in our analysis of the interview transcripts: (1) being normal through work and men; (2) disclosure for better or worse; (3) care work; (4) caring for violent men; and (4) women's bodies. Sometimes these mirror the dominant discourse, sometimes they pose alternative resistance discourses, and always they reveal the tensions and links between oppression and resistance. The five discourses identified illustrate how women draw upon discourses of femininity and normalcy as ways of reconstructing themselves as humans in the face of dominant discourses that identify HIV-positive women as something less than human. All five share an overarching core feature of wrestling with the problem of stigma and using notions and practices of femininity to attempt to overcome stigma and appear normal and acceptable. Within each discourse, however, we also found ambiguity, contradiction, and resistance. At the same time the women were attempting to appear "normal," they also questioned and sometimes even challenged these constructs of femininity and normalcy.

Analysis of Qualitative Data

The intent of our research was to examine the ways in which the dominant discourses described in the HIV literature by scholars such as Seidel (1993) are disclosed in how women living with HIV in a marginalized population in a Cape Town support group describe their lives. The discourses Seidel describes are discussed in depth in the next chapter. The discourses identified in our research emerge from the "talk" that took place between the researcher and the participants. Talk, as in the talk that takes place in an interview, can be taken at face value. For example, one reason we chose to interview women living with HIV is that it is our belief that these women's voices are not heard and that their opinions and needs are often not reflected in policy that governs how they are treated. Their experiences and opinions are invisible in the ways issues surrounding HIV are identified, assessed, and addressed in society (Bell, 2005). Recording and describing their experiences and ideas, therefore, was essential to our research, but it was not sufficient. If we were to do a thematic analysis of our interviews, we would stop at just reporting the answers our participants gave to the questions we asked them and would analyze them by considering how their answers related to their social context. Because we were particularly interested in the politics of the ways in which the women in our study experience HIV, we chose to take another step in the analysis and proceed to a critical discourse analysis.

Discourse analysis allowed us to explore the political dimensions of the social context in which the women in our study are living with HIV. We were able to see, for example, how dominant discourses about women's bodies, which are part of the politics of gender that identify women as other and problematize women's bodies, create challenges for women living with the physical changes that stem from HIV and ARVs. In addition to seeing the importance of dominant discourse and the power that systems of inequality have over people's lives, we also were able to identify challenges to these systems in alternative discourses that the women have constructed in order to reject ideals that degrade them.

Naples (2003) writes that her research shows that "discourse is not the property of individual actors or social movement organizations" (p. 106). In fact, it is possible for women to create their own counter discourses in response to or in addition to the dominant ones, and this is necessary because these counter discourses have material consequences in the possible furthering of the agenda of the women themselves (Naples 2003).

During our interviews and through our analysis of the transcripts of the conversations with the women, it became apparent that there were important messages lying beneath the surface. Critical discourse analysis allowed us to read between the lines. Peeking beneath the conversations, we found that the women interviewed are indeed affected by the dominant discourses identified in the literature on the gendered aspects of HIV that have been written about them. More importantly, however, the women did not exclusively draw upon the discourses apparent in the scholarly literature to describe their experience. Nor did they cite the primary issues that had been identified in the literature as their main concerns. Instead, as Foucault (1978) and Naples (2003) predict, the women have created their own discourses about themselves, and these are discourses of femininity, normalization, and resistance.

4 Marginalizing the Marginalized through Multiple Stigmas

AIDS is a war against humanity. We need to break the silence, banish the stigma and discrimination and ensure total inclusiveness within the struggle against AIDS. If we discard the people living with HIV/AIDS, we can no longer call ourselves human.

Nelson Mandela

MOST SCHOLARS AND activists now recognize stigma as one of the most important factors in the lives of people living with HIV (Mahajan et al., 2008). There is no escaping the stigma that is attached to HIV. Everyone who is living with HIV is stigmatized to some extent. The experiences of that stigma, however, fluctuate across many variables, including gender. Women and men are stigmatized differently—for example, there are differences in regard to the extent to which men and women are blamed for their actions that supposedly led to their HIV-positive status. The blaming that occurs in HIV stigma is linked to gender and reproductive roles that define "good" and "bad" behavior and "wrongdoings," especially sexual "misbehaviors," which are different for men and women. Most women are still held to a double standard that expects them to be less interested in sex and more responsible for controlling both their own sexual behavior and that of their men partners (Lorber & Moore, 2002).

Furthermore, the staying power or escalation of gendered HIV stigma may stem from the fact that stigmatization in general is inextricably linked to a marginalization or "othering" of one kind or another, and gender "others" women. In societies where masculine hegemony exists, women are marginalized. Women are compared negatively to norms where masculinity is considered the normal, correct, superior model. Women, then, are deemed as not behaving properly as women if they stray from the prescribed formulas of femininity. Or if women are properly feminine, then they are not as intelligent, strong, or valuable as men and not quite human, since men are the measure of humanity. HIV stigmatization, therefore, adds to the "normal" marginalization of women.

What Is Gendered HIV Stigma?

In order to understand the many aspects of HIV stigma, it is helpful to understand how stigma has been described. Goffman (1963), one of the first scholars to study stigma, explained it as the belief that "people who possess a characteristic defined as socially undesirable acquire a 'spoiled identity' which then leads to social devaluation and discrimination" (p. 15). His definition notes the relationship between stigma and discrimination. When people with supposedly undesirable traits are stigmatized, it is likely that they are also discriminated against. This two-step process has been observed in the perception and treatment of people who are living with HIV, and Goffman's definition remains the dominant one in research on the virus. In their HIV stigma research for the Human Sciences Research Council (HSRC) in South Africa, for example, Deacon, Stephney, and Prosalendis (2005) discuss the distinction between stigma and discrimination and the link between the two terms. They define "HIV stigma" as negative ideas about people living with HIV, and "discrimination" as the actions that are taken that unfairly disadvantage those people.

Other aspects of Goffman's work on stigma have been altered in contemporary thinking about HIV. He and other classical theorists focused their attention on the micro-interactions among individuals and did not link stigma to the larger social context. More recent scholars, however, have expanded upon Goffman's ideas and now understand stigma as a political issue. They observe that stigma does not take place within a vacuum; rather, it occurs within social contexts that include political relationships, inequities, and tensions. Stigma is influenced by this context and serves to maintain existing power relations ensuring that those who are perceived as "others" are kept in that position. In addition, not just relationships of inequity but systems of inequality themselves are retained in part by the use of stigma (Deacon et al., 2005). Stigma and subsequent discrimination "[have] the effect of reproducing relations of social inequality that are advantageous to the dominant class, [thus] these forms of stigmatisation are functional [at least for those in positions of power] in the sense that they help maintain the socio-political status quo" (p. 17). Stigma directs any social critique toward individuals who do not fit properly within the existing system of social relations rather than toward the system itself. Stigma focuses attention on the supposed failings of individuals and groups of people and away from the inequalities and failings of the social systems in which they interact.

In the case of HIV, stigma is a powerful othering force that has an impact on who gets blamed for the disease, who is allowed access to treatment, and how people living with the virus experience their lives and themselves. HIV stigma sorts people into "good" people, those who are not HIV positive, and "bad" people, those who are living with HIV. In addition, the stigma justifies the scarcity of treatments available and the rationing of the resources. Stigma, then, is a political tool that helps to maintain the status quo by ensuring that only certain people—those in less powerful positions—are blamed for problems such as the emergence and spread of the HI virus, and that existing relations of power are kept in place. Since gender is a system of power, stigmatizing women who are living with HIV is both a useful ideological tool to fortify existing gendered power relations as well as an ideological tool to marginalize people living with HIV.

Stigmatizing Beliefs about Women Living with HIV

Seidel (1993) has studied how HIV/AIDS discourse, the way in which society talks about HIV, can contribute to stigma. She speaks about several discourses that operate in sub-Saharan Africa regarding HIV, including developmental, legal, ethical, activist, medical, and medico-moral discourses. Developmental discourse refers to the discussion of HIV as a barrier to development in the Global South. As such, it becomes a key item on the agenda in relationships between North and South nations and legitimizes the intervention of the North in Southern nations around issues related to HIV (Kole, 2008). This kind of discourse presents HIV as an economic barrier to Southern nations, as it prevents these nations from successfully increasing their gross domestic product. Discussions center on the lost productivity of workers who are ill. The solution to the problem in this discourse is to rely on the experts and resources of the Global North to address HIV at the same time they offer remedies to what they see as the economic failings of the Global South. In developmental discourse, people living with HIV are conceptualized as inefficient workers, the Global South is perceived as an inefficient economic manager, and the Global North is seen as a role model for improvement.

A second discourse is the legal discourse, which is most concerned with the legal rights of people infected and affected by HIV, such as guaranteeing confidentiality and protecting their privacy. This way of thinking and speaking about HIV represents people living with the virus as citizens of various nations whose civil rights need to be protected. One area of concern, for example, has been the legal rights of children to continue in school after they have been diagnosed as HIV positive (Blumenreich, 2003).

The ethical discourse perceives HIV as one of the major ethical issues facing humanity today and addresses the need to seek the best solutions for the common good by balancing science and medicine with other concerns, such as the right to privacy or the right to refuse medical diagnosis (testing) or treatment. It focuses on ethical principles in the treatment of people living with HIV and calls attention to the ethical problems of a world where people do not have adequate access to health care. For example, Gillies (2004), a proponent of this point of view, writes, "Scientific knowledge should be made available to all who can benefit from it; individualism should be put into the context of the common good; and free market forces need to be modified to reflect the fact that we live in a world that is increasingly interdependent" (p. 284).

The activist discourse presents HIV as a political issue and highlights the activities, motivations, and impact of HIV activism on political, economic, social, and ideological debates around HIV (Mbali, 2005). While the activist discourse overlaps with the ethical and legal discourses, it goes a step further by suggesting that the reason we face these ethical and legal issues is because of political structures and relationships that prevent our being able to act in the most ethical ways and to establish and promote the human and civil rights necessary to protect people living with HIV. In chapter 3 we described the point of view of the TAC as representing the activist discourse, a viewpoint we share. Seidel asserts that while all of these can be found in discussions of HIV in media, scholarly forums, and political arenas, two other discourses are most prominent in the creation of HIV stigma: the medical and the medico-moral discourses. Medical discourse refers to messages from large medical authorities such as the World Health Organization (WHO) that emphasize the medical condition of people living with HIV and reduce humans to symptoms, stages, and blood counts. Besides this dehumanizing of HIV-positive people, the medical discourse has invented terms like "high-risk group" that end up stigmatizing people who are identified with particular groups within a society. The term "high-risk group" refers to highly studied (when it comes to the HIV pandemic) communities of people, such as gay men and men who have sex with men, people of color, intravenous drug users, and sex workers. Women are also one such group. Referring to women as high risk stigmatizes and others all women, but it has especially identified women of color in low-income communities of the Global South. When women are referred to as a high-risk group and they are members of specific, already marginalized communities, it appears that there is a unique elevated rate or risk of HIV infection coming from something within particular groups of people. In contrast, other groups of people who are not marginalized, such as heterosexual men or white people in general, are thought of and talked about as not at high risk and therefore supposedly not intrinsically prone to HIV. In reality, however, actual risk is associated with particular behaviors, not specific communities of people. Yet the discourse identifies certain groups as high risk, thereby allowing them to be blamed for their own infection and for the spread of infection into the dominant "innocent" groups of people.

The medico-moral discourse is a further extension of the medical model. Based on the premise of the medical model of "high-risk groups," the medico-moral discourse presents people living with HIV as morally depraved and blames them for the bad behavior that caused them to become HIV positive. The medico-moral discourse is represented, for example, by right-wing Christian groups who claim that AIDS is God's punishment on humans who do not abide by his laws (Seidel, 1993).

Stigmatization by Medical and Medico-Moral Discourses about HIV in the Global South

Many people have been categorized as "other" and subsequently stigmatized in this way in HIV-related discourses. In addition to gender, social class, sexuality, and race ethnicity, another important category is nation or region. For example, the term "Pattern II countries," widely used among scholars and policy makers, including powerful agencies such as the National Institutes of Health (NIH) and Centers for Disease Control (CDC) in the United States, creates stigma through their construction of "African AIDS" (Seidel, 1993, p. 177). This terminology makes it appear as if the virus manifests itself as a completely different and exceptionally virulent type of disease on the continent of Africa as opposed to the "safer," more "normal" type of HIV found in North America and Europe. The use of such terms leads to the stigmatization of both HIV-positive and non-positive people living in Africa. It also furthers the racist way in which black and/or African sexualities have been constructed by the Global North as "primitive" and "deviant" (Austin, 1989; Collins, 2004). And the stigma is endorsed by the authoritative voices of scientific health-care professionals. The linked stigmas of racism, sexual stereotypes, and national prejudice that operate in medical discourses "have profound implications for funding and for international solidarity. It is a new, very authoritative and sophisticated variety of the discourse of control and exclusion, which, because of its medical and scientific stable, passes as neutral and non-ideological" (Seidel, 1993, p. 177).

This multiple layering of stigma has brought together various social categories such as region and sexuality and serves to intensify the othering of those who are in more than one marginalized group (Ratele & Shefer, 2002). The myths about who started the AIDS pandemic present an example of these multiple layers of stigmatization. The myths also present examples of how stigma is not just an ideological problem but can lead to differential treatment of marginalized people. In the United States, AIDS mythology maintains that HIV was initially identified in gay men. This supposed link between a disease and gay men fueled homophobia and the idea that AIDS was a disease that would punish the "atrocity" of gay sexuality (Ratele & Shefer, 2002).

A parallel but contrasting myth in the United States maintains that the beginnings of the pandemic mysteriously started in Haitian people, which subsequently led to the belief by the CDC that Haitians were inherently and inexplicably susceptible to HIV infection. The promotion of this belief by such a high-profile scientific organization led to the resulting quarantine and detention of Haitian immigrants (and anyone "resembling" a Haitian immigrant) in the United States (Farmer, 1992; Sessions, 2001). The CDC has since disclaimed this idea, but the Haitian story continues to both draw on and reinforce the racist link between ideas about sexual deviance and promiscuity and being black (Collins, 2000).

And there is, of course, the theory that AIDS started in Africa as a result of humans coming into close physical contact with monkeys infected with simian immunodeficiency virus (SIV), a virus similar to the human immunodeficiency virus that purportedly crossed species and mutated into what we now know as HIV (Chirimuuta & Chirimuuta, 1989; Gallo, 2006). This story galvanizes the global racist assumptions about the continent of Africa and of black people in general as having "untamed" or deviant sexual practices. Over the years, these ideas regarding othered or marginalized groups of people that fueled the pandemic has led to the subsequent stigmatization of sex workers, drug users, and, in general, poor women of color, especially those who live in Africa.

In addition to these global stories fueling stigmatization of people who are HIV positive, local beliefs have created stories that supplement them. According to a study by Kalichman and Simbayi (2004), a particular stigma surrounding people living with HIV occurs in several South African townships and other rural areas on the continent that stems from traditional supernatural beliefs. Some South Africans believe that the Ancestors and God send illness or withdraw protection from illness because a person has done something bad in their life. Illness is seen as an indicator of wrongdoing, and, therefore, the person should be considered dirty and should be ashamed and avoided. This particular type of stigma is also present on the other side of the globe as part of the fundamentalist-Christian myth in the United States that claims HIV is "God's punishment" for being gay (Seidel, 1993).

In all of these cases, a powerful myth has been generated that identifies certain categories of people as supposedly susceptible to AIDS. We, of course, do not know when and where HIV first affected humans. We do know, on the other hand, that the spread of HIV is associated with certain behaviors in which all humans engage regardless of their skin color, the sex of their partner, or where they make their home on the planet. But the stories about the origins of HIV and who is "high risk," and therefore who is supposedly not at risk, serve to perpetuate existing systems of stigmatization and discrimination.

Stigma and Blame

Alongside the stigmatization of all of these categories by race, nation, sexuality, and occupation is the stigma of gender. Women have been characterized as having played an important role in causing and spreading HIV. Over the years, women have been directly and indirectly referred to as vectors of HIV. Women being constructed as vectors appears in the programs that have been established in attempts to slow the spread of the virus. According to Seidel (1993), conservative Christian groups often establish HIV education and intervention programs that serve to further stigmatize women by holding them accountable for the spread of the virus. Interventions that center on the value of chastity, abstinence, and staying faithful (the ABCs we describe in chapter 1), for example, focus on women as gatekeepers for sexuality. These programs have been promoted all over the world, including South Africa.

In addition, communities in South Africa have created other interventions such as virginity testing, where girls and young women are "tested" for their virginity by older women community members (Hoosen & Collins, 2004). It is thought that if these girls and young women pass the test, they will be empowered to abstain from sex before marriage, curbing the spread of HIV. Virginity testing has been strongly condemned by the South African government and is now banned for girls under the age of 16, because it poses a human rights violation against girls and young women (Children's Act, 2005). Furthermore, virginity testing approaches do not test for HIV, and they place all the blame and responsibility for the spread of the virus in the hands of women and girls. Virginity testing is still part of an ongoing debate in many areas in South Africa; however, it is not widely accepted. Other, more common practices, such as advocating placing more control of HIV prevention in the hands of women—for example, through the use of microbicides and female condoms—face similar problems. Mantell and her colleagues (2006), for example, assert that the result of the introduction of women-controlled methods of HIV prevention has been a paradox in that the same structures that are barriers to HIV prevention in women (such as lack of control over their own sexuality and lack of power to shape their partner's behavior, which we described in our discussion of the limitations of ABCs) also preclude acceptance of these methods. So even when the burden of responsibility of prevention is unfairly placed on women, it is still impossible for women to exert real control over the matter. Furthermore, studies of the sexual practices of young adults in South Africa show that, as in many places in the world, boys and young men are encouraged to have numerous sexual experiences as a "natural" part of manhood (Reddy, 2005). These ideas of "natural" conduct for men and "good" conduct for women create stigma for women living with HIV, because they endorse the idea that women who "misbehave" wind up HIV positive and spread the virus to others.

Another way that women have been constructed as vectors of HIV is through the idea of reproductive responsibility. In their study of women's experiences of stigma, Lekas, Siegel, and Schrimshaw (2006) report that HIV-positive women experience intense stigma from the medical community and society as a whole if they choose to have children. Women in their study felt they were being punished for having become infected, because they were discouraged from becoming mothers, despite the fact that there are now effective ARV measures available to women who are HIV positive and want to have children who are HIV negative. This kind of stigma becomes even more problematic in the context of South Africa, because studies have shown that women's fertility is associated with a positive social status (Cooper et al., 2007; Strebel, 1995). Being HIV positive and childless is a double blow to some women, because it exacerbates their position as other.

Stigmatizing and Social Distancing

Blame is not the only form of stigmatization. Social distancing is also important. Adam and Sears (1996) found that women living with HIV have a unique set of problems that isolates them from the rest of society. This isolation begins in the form of beliefs within a society or a certain community about women living with the virus. For example, isolation occurs when family and community members express a fear of being in contact with women who are HIV positive, lest they become infected. This form of distancing is illustrated by family members physically separating themselves from those who are HIV positive and taking excessive precautions to disinfect items the person has come into contact with. Lekas and her colleagues (2006) refer to these kinds of behaviors as "hygienic degradation acts" (p. 1180), including separating eating utensils, clothing, and cosmetics as well as keeping a distance from people living with HIV for fear of contagion. Such behaviors are documented in numerous studies on HIV and stigma and stem, in part, from persistent erroneous beliefs people have about HIV transmission (Castle, 2004; Lekas et al., 2006; Li et al., 2006).

Hoosen and Collins (2004) point out that although most research claims that the majority of people are now aware of the true routes of HIV transmission, strong evidence exists to suggest otherwise. In their research in South Africa, they found that some people in their study were unsure about or inaccurate in their knowledge of HIV transmission; there were even those who claimed to have never heard of condoms. A lack of basic HIV knowledge shows up again in the research done by Castle (2004) in Mali. In her study, Castle spoke to children, teachers, leaders, and parents in a community about HIV stigma. She found that children and parents especially, and teachers and leaders to some extent, exhibit "great confusion" (p. 6) about how the virus is transmitted. Their beliefs ranged from thinking that the infection is spread by defecating and urinating in the same place as others, to thinking that HIV started when girls were paid to have sex with white people's dogs. These beliefs go hand in hand with the beliefs that people living with HIV are dirty and disgusting and should be avoided.

The beliefs are also linked to ideas about sexuality that cast people who are HIV positive as extraordinarily and immorally engaged in sex. Castle found that the children in her study felt that HIV-positive people should be separated from society and deserved little compassion. By having sexual relations, people living with the virus were viewed as having transgressed social norms that emphasize abstinence before marriage or faithfulness within it. Those who were HIV positive were therefore perceived as having broken the rule and thereby brought the illness upon themselves. This attitude especially stigmatizes women living with HIV as another piece of this set of social norms that holds women most responsible for chastity and faithfulness in marriage.

Women's Experiences of Stigma

HIV stigma is complex and layered in the way that it is experienced and can ultimately lead to lost opportunities, social isolation, and the internalization of stigmatizing ideas (Fife & Wright, 2000). A person living with the virus may have personal experiences of being stigmatized, or she may have been outright discriminated against because of her status. People can also perceive stigma when they witness discrimination against others living with the virus (Lekas et al., 2006). In any case, these stigmatizing experiences, along with experiences and beliefs a person may have had prior to testing positive for HIV, are likely to lead to internalization (Fife & Wright, 2000).

Internal stigma, also known as felt stigma, self-stigmatization, and perceived stigma, has been identified in the literature as an aspect of HIV stigma (Deacon et al., 2005; Lekas et al., 2006; Visser, Makin & Lehobye, 2006). There is some debate as to how these terms should be conceptualized in regard to whether they are types of internal stigma or "linked processes" of internal stigmatization (Deacon et al., 2005, p. 21). Nevertheless, they can be understood as the process by which people living with HIV start to believe the negative ideas about individuals who are HIV positive. These beliefs may come in the form of the internalization of negative feelings about contracting the virus, feeling ashamed, and condemning themselves for their own sexual practices or misfortunes and the harm that the virus is causing in their lives. In addition, internal stigma may lead people to believe that because they are HIV positive, they are unclean, bad, and are being punished for their "careless behavior" (Nyblade, 2006).

Self-stigmatization is even more of a problem for women because of the abundance of stigmatizing beliefs surrounding women's sexuality (Lorber & Moore, 2002). These include the notions of good women being sexually passive and the perpetuation of the racist link between sexual promiscuity and blackness, even without the added factor of being HIV positive (Collins, 2000; 2004). In addition, women may internalize HIV stigma because of the discourse of women as vectors who are responsible for spreading the disease (Ratele & Shefer, 2002). Their perceived reproductive roles cast women who are HIV positive and have children as vertical vectors of the virus in mother-to-child transmission (Lekas et al., 2006; Visser et al., 2006).

Internal stigmatization is a serious problem because of the psychological pain it causes the individual. It is especially detrimental to women living with HIV, because it can prevent them from seeking help in the forms of social and medical support and quite possibly leads to their punishing themselves for having become HIV positive (Fife & Wright, 2000).

Stigma and Disclosure of HIV-Positive Status

When a person receives a positive result on an HIV test, she or he faces the dilemma of whether or not to tell anyone. Disclosure is an important issue because it may determine whether a person seeks treatment (Klitzman et al., 2004). In order to receive treatment (if it is available at all), people must, at the very least, disclose their status to health-care workers. Disclosure must also take place in order for a person living with HIV to receive social, emotional, and adherence to treatment support (Klitzman et al., 2004). The literature shows that stigma is oftentimes an insurmountable barrier to disclosure, especially for women. However, this is not always true, and some research shows that stigma may not necessarily be a barrier to preventing women from taking care of their health.

Women in Burkina Faso, like many women all over the world, have weak economic status, low levels of education, begin having sex with older men at an early age, rarely use condoms, and are submissive to men. Despite these constraints, a study by Issiaka and her colleagues (2001) shows that most women living with HIV say that their number-one concern is their health. This suggests that they are more concerned with their health than they are with the tasks of disclosing their status and dealing with stigma. The women living with HIV in the study who at first decided not to disclose and then changed their mind said their primary fear was that their partner would reject or abandon them or think they had been unfaithful. However, upon disclosure, the most common reaction from partners was that of indifference. In other words, stigma in Burkina Faso was not as important as the women had feared, and in their own view of their HIV status, health problems were more important than being stigmatized.

Research in the United States shows similar findings. Kimberly, Serovich, and Greene (1995) examined case histories of women living with HIV who had already disclosed their status to friends and family. Some of the women said they were not so much concerned with stigma as they were with the personal situations of the recipients of their disclosures. Other women in the study wanted to delay disclosure to their mothers, because their mothers were suffering from their own illnesses and the women did not want to upset them. While some of the women in these studies did not find stigma to be a large barrier to disclosure, other women living with HIV do.

Many of the women in the Burkina Faso study by Issiaka and her colleagues (2001) did express that stigma was indeed a barrier to disclosure. The women in this study who did not disclose were worried about rejection, abandonment, being accused of being unfaithful, and withdrawal of financial support from family members, who may not want to invest money in someone whom they believe is going to die soon. Some women were worried about a reaction of violence, even though the women in the Burkina Faso study did not report violent reactions from men partners as other women have in the United States, Kenya, South Africa, and Rwanda (Rothenberg, 1995; Seidel & Ntuli, 1996; Temmerman, 1995; Van der Straten, King, Grinstead, Serufilira & Allen, 1995). Several women in the study by Kimberly and her colleagues (1995) disclosed only to close friends and family for fear of being fired, being evicted, losing health insurance, or losing custody of their children. In summary, making the decision to disclose is not easy, because it is difficult to gauge the type and extent of the stigma, discrimination, rejection, and punishment that one may experience as a result. The research across several nations shows most significantly that women carefully weigh a broad and complex array of possible consequences in order to make the determination of what to do next (Serovich, 2001). As we shall see in chapter 5, the process of decision making about disclosure in the context of all the various forms of stigma is an extraordinary challenge.

The Psychological Impact of Stigma on Women Living with HIV

There are psychological implications of stigma whether a woman is experiencing self-stigma, stigma in a community, or stigma by a social institution. It is essential to look at the psychological problems that HIV-positive people experience because of the human suffering caused by emotional reactions to stigma. But "psychological processes" also contribute to worsening physical health in people who are living with HIV (Brief et al., 2004, p. 6). Furthermore, the link between social stigma, psychological manifestations of the stress induced by the stigma, and increased physical health problems appears to be exacerbated in women. For example, the higher presence of symptoms of depression among those living with the virus may be associated with a higher level of morbidity and mortality for women who are HIV positive than for men who are HIV positive (Hader, Smith, Moore & Holmberg, 2001). At the very least, the mental health effects of living with HIV lead to a poorer quality of life and will worsen the experiences of women, who are already a marginalized community (Lorber & Moore, 2002; Tostes, Chalub & Botega, 2004).

According to Fife and Wright (2000), people living with HIV in the United States experience more feelings of stigmatization than people with other serious illnesses, such as cancer. In addition, among the HIV-positive people in their study, women experienced even more feelings of stigmatization than did men. Fife and Wright claim that women feel more social isolation because they have less support due to their fear of the consequences of disclosure, which are more likely to affect them—for example, losing custody of their children. Because of this isolation, women end up internalizing these feelings, which results in poorer self-esteem. Similarly, in Brazil, women who are living with HIV are more likely than men to experience symptoms of depression resulting from stigma. The social consequences of HIV coupled with the marginal status of women in general means that women are especially at risk for psychological problems that result from living with HIV (Tostes et al., 2004).

Stigma Is a Barrier to Maintaining Health for Women Living with HIV

Probably the most important step a woman who is HIV positive, or is in danger of becoming HIV positive, can take for herself is to pay attention to her physical health. This means being able to access and use condoms and avoiding situations where sexual violence or coercion are possibilities. These may sound like relatively basic steps, but according to the literature, stigma often stands in the way of women who are trying to attain these goals.

Seidel (1993) states that in many countries the medico-moral discourse dominates. For example, large numbers of people believe that making condoms available to women encourages promiscuity, and therefore it is considered taboo for women to even discuss condom use. Not only the general public but governments too have bought into this discourse. In Ghana condoms are available for some women, but women who have condoms or ask their partner to use one may be seen as "loose" or "dirty" (Mill & Anarfi, 2002). When there is a stigma against women using condoms, it is difficult for women to protect themselves against becoming infected or being repeatedly reinfected with HIV or other sexually transmitted infections. Examples like these can be found in nearly every nation in the world. Uganda represents a particularly clear example of the medico-moral discourse in action, where the message is coming from the collaboration of two nations: Uganda and the United States.

Uganda is one of the focus nations of the PEPFAR (President's Emergency Plan for AIDS Relief) program. PEPFAR is the centerpiece of the U.S. government's global health initiative and is engaged in developing and funding an international aid program for addressing the problem of HIV. In 2005 under the Bush administration, PEPFAR issued formal guidelines for countries that were receiving funds from the U.S. government for AIDS work. The guidelines included a number of highly controversial restrictions. First, PEPFAR required that prevention programs emphasize the AB of the ABC program: Abstinence only and Be faithful. Although funding was also provided for condoms, they were restricted in programs with young people under the age of 24 and those who were unmarried. Condoms could not be distributed in schools and could only be provided to young people who were considered to be in high-risk groups. In addition, although campaigns directed toward high-risk youth were allowed to mention condoms, such campaigns were required to emphasize abstinence and being faithful. The guidelines state: "Implementing partners must take great care not to give a conflicting message with regard to abstinence by confusing abstinence messages with condom marketing campaigns that appear to encourage sexual activity or appear to present abstinence and condom use as equally viable, alternative choices. Thus, marketing campaigns that target youth and encourage condom use as the primary intervention are not appropriate for youth, and the Emergency Plan will not fund them" (PEPFAR, 2005, p. 32). The regulation required that at least a third of the funds for prevention be earmarked for AB programs. The programs were highly successful in adhering to the regulations, and in 2005 that quota was surpassed, with 56 percent of the funds for prevention from PEPFAR going to AB programs.

Even in programs when the PEPFAR regulations do not restrict the distribution of condoms, they have created confusion and fear that has resulted in organizations constraining their work in order to eliminate condom campaigns and other reproductive health programs. Research by the Center for Strategic and International Studies (Fleischman, 2006) reports: "There are perceived restrictions in PEPFAR about what you can discuss with whom, so everyone is being very cautious. . . . People are afraid to discuss family planning, condoms, abortion—so many groups don't address them at all" (p. 23). In Zambia, for example, because program implementers believed that these measures were required by PEPFAR, several PEPFAR-funded organizations not only stopped promoting condoms but also eliminated any reference to condoms in their programs for fear that they would lose their funding (SIECUS, 2009).

The requirement that 33 percent of funds for prevention be spent on AB work was lifted in 2008 when PEPFAR renewed funding for HIV organizations. Unfortunately, condom distribution is still prohibited for individuals under age 16, even though these very young people are at risk for HIV. In addition, organizations must send Congress a report "if less than half of prevention funds go to abstinence, delay of sexual debut, monogamy, fidelity and partner reduction in any host country with a generalized epidemic" (Office of the Law Revision Counsel, 2010).

A second controversial guideline required programs receiving PEPFAR funds to take an anti-prostitution pledge, which obligated them to sign a promise stating that they opposed prostitution in order to receive funding. PEPFAR rules in 2003 stated: "No funds made available to carry out this Act, or any amendment made by this Act, may be used to provide assistance to any group or organization that does not have a policy explicitly opposing prostitution and sex trafficking" (Avert, 2005). Many organizations that had worked with commercial sex workers for years refused to sign the pledge, because they believed it would make the sex workers uncertain about where their loyalties were and would therefore hinder the ability of organizations to continue their work—for example, of distributing condoms to sex workers. The Brazilian government and the BBC World Service turned down millions of dollars in funding because they did not feel they could carry out their work under the restriction. In 2011 a U.S. Federal Appeals Court ruled that the pledge was not legal and could not be required of programs seeking funding.

A third controversial piece of the PEPFAR program is the "conscience clause," which allows organizations that receive U.S. funds for AIDS work

> to choose those groups and individuals to whom they are "morally" comfortable providing care, thereby permitting the denial of services to those whose behavior, identity, religion, or other attributes may be deemed unacceptable. During the nearly three decades of the HIV/AIDS epidemic, efforts to reduce and eliminate stigmatization of those infected and those at risk have been a critical factor in successful approaches to prevention. Yet, the conscience

> clause actually codifies the acceptance of stigmatization and discrimination and allows the use of U.S. taxpayer funds to perpetuate such discrimination. (PEPFARWatch, 2008, p. 1)

In addition to creating discrimination and stigmatization, the conscience clause also interferes with offering the best information and materials for HIV prevention to those who are served by organizations that are ideologically opposed to such information—for example, discussions of male and female condoms.

Initially PEPFAR supporters presented Uganda as an exemplary nation when the numbers of people living with HIV fell in the first years of the twenty-first century. More recently, however, reports are showing that in 2012 Uganda is one of only two nations (along with Mali) in Africa where the number of new cases of HIV is increasing. Some critics are now saying that Uganda's partnership with PEPFAR and conservative religious organizations may have "merely succeeded in driving certain behaviors further underground in this socially conservative country with close ties to American evangelicals" (Kron, 2012, p. 1). For example, one survey conducted in Uganda found that although 90 percent of Ugandans acknowledge sexual fidelity in a relationship as a health imperative, about 25 percent of married men said they had multiple sexual partners. The research also found that while 75 percent of Ugandans were knowledgeable about condoms in sexual health, fewer than 8 percent of married men who were having sex outside their marriage were using condoms. One religious leader and AIDS activist explained, "If you have an environment that stigmatizes them, then don't expect people to use condoms" (Kron, 2012, p.1). In the case of Uganda, the medico-moral discourse has stigmatized the use of condoms and the nation has been left with a collapse in HIV prevention.

Finding Alternative Discourses in the Fight against HIV

HIV stigma is a force that creates barriers against accessing proper support and health care for people living with HIV. It is not only an outside force, but it is also a force from within, meaning many people must battle with their own internal stigma, especially women, who must deal with a particularly gendered form of HIV stigma. HIV stigma is especially powerful and debilitating because it is linked to other forms of stigmatization. Multiple layers of stigma and discrimination push women living with HIV even further to the margins. How do women respond? What tools do they use to fend off stigmatization and to bring themselves "back to normal"?

In the next five chapters we address these questions by identifying and describing the major discourses that emerged in interviews with women who are living with HIV in Cape Town, South Africa. In this chapter we have reviewed some of the dominant discourses among policy makers, medical professionals, and governmental officials. The marginalized women we will meet in the next five chapters reveal discourse around HIV that are quite different from the dominant discourses identified by Seidel (1993).

The five discourses that emerged in our analysis of the interview transcripts are: (1) disclosure for better or worse; (2) being normal through work and intimate relationships with men; (3) care work for children; (4) caring for violent men, even in the face of abuse; and (5) the appearance of women's bodies. These five discourses illustrate how women draw upon discourses of femininity and normalcy as ways of reconstructing themselves as humans in the face of dominant discourses that identify HIV-positive women as something less than human.

The overarching theme that emerges in these interviews and draws these five issues together is that of women striving to be what they believe, or what they think we or others hearing them speak believe, is "normal." For these women, the struggle to be or to seem normal has been accomplished (or not) through emphasized femininity. Women draw on hegemonic gender expectations in these discourses, which are explored in the following chapters.

5 Disclosure for Better or Worse

FOR THOSE WHO are HIV positive, disclosure is an essential step. If nothing else, they must at least disclose their status to health-care providers in order to obtain care and medicine. Disclosure also contributes to a person's ability to take care of themselves and to plan ahead for their care and treatment. However, disclosure is not easy. Telling others that one is HIV positive is always difficult and sometimes impossible. The stigma associated with the virus creates a monumental problem. Not surprisingly, in our interviews with HIV-positive women, a significant discourse emerged around the issue of disclosure.

The decision to disclose one's HIV status and the process of then doing so are constant worries for the women we interviewed, and their conversations with us revealed their dilemmas and decisions regarding disclosure in myriad ways. Three main areas seemed most salient: (1) disclosing at work and the favorable and unfavorable consequences of doing so; (2) disclosing to children and mothers of the women, particularly the issue of fearing their reactions; and (3) disclosing to acquaintances who are not well known or even complete strangers as a way of seeking acknowledgment for being a survivor and activist and as a way of following the advice of medical and psychological authorities.

The best way to illustrate the operation of the discourse of disclosure is to look at some specific instances in which women speak about it. As we saw in the previous chapter, the medical discourse and the activist discourse present very different views of HIV and the people who live with it. These two points of view, however, share at least one idea, and that is the importance of disclosure. Both medical professionals and HIV activists encourage women and men to reveal their status publicly. People who are HIV positive are encouraged and sometimes even required to disclose their status as a way to improve public health and to improve their own mental and physical health. This point of view is based on the assumption of the "talking cure," which is the foundation of the discipline of psychology and psychotherapy—a discourse of the dominant medical establishment. HIV activists also promote disclosure, although for somewhat different reasons. They too believe that disclosure is useful for addressing self-stigmatization. But they also advocate disclosure as a way to challenge stigmatization and discrimination against people living with HIV by those who believe that the virus is a problem of others unlike themselves. The women in our study are aware of the positions of both the medical profession and the activist community regarding disclosure and have given it careful consideration. However, from the point of view and experience of the women we interviewed, disclosure is seen as a step that may or may not always be absolutely positive or the best one for them to take. In the next section we look at what these women said about HIV disclosure and some of the meanings behind their comments.

Disclosure in the Workplace

One of the participants in our research who spoke about revealing her HIV status is Elaine. Elaine has disclosed her status at work and at the weekly HIV support group meetings, and she frequently talked about the problems that have resulted or could result from disclosing. For example, throughout our interview Elaine mentioned problems with the management at the factory where she works. She talked about work as she described the day she first tested positive for HIV. On this same day she was required to attend a mandatory meeting with several members of management regarding her repeated absences from work.

> The meeting was too heavy and they didn't want to listen to me, so I took out the letter [her HIV-positive diagnosis from the clinic] and I was crying. . . . Then they said to me, "What's wrong with you Elaine?" I said to them, "No, I just found out now that I'm HIV positive and I didn't wanted to tell you." They say, "WHAT? Is it really true?" I give them the letter. . . . They said to me, "How did you find out?" I said, "No, I went to the clinic and the doctor asked me to do an HIV test, so I did the test and my test came out I am HIV positive." And they said to me, "Okay, Elaine we can't fire you now. We don't have to fire you."

The fact that Elaine was forced to disclose her HIV status—quite possibly a person's most intimate secret—is an illustration of how all-powerful a workplace is for a person. She was forced to choose between her personal privacy and her job. Fortunately for Elaine, this disclosure, although painful, may have given her some peace of mind in terms of job security, because South African law demands that employers do not discriminate against employees who are HIV positive (Department of Labour Employment Equity Act, 1998). This is no small benefit in a country, much less a world, where job security is rare and where jobs are a lifeline to survival as well as a defining part of ourselves.

The current rate of unemployment in South Africa is about 24.8 percent and about 23.8 percent in the Western Cape, where Cape Town is located (Bloomberg Brief, 2012; Statistics South Africa, 2012). The area where Elaine and the other women we interviewed live is somewhat removed from the Cape Town city center and therefore separated from many job opportunities. In her community the people who have found work are often employed at one of a few factories. These few factories have their pick of employees, hiring and firing as they please, because the number of people searching for work far outnumbers the positions available. When management at the factory where Elaine works found out that she was HIV positive, they were legally restrained by South African laws from firing her, even if they were disturbed by her disclosure and by the days she had missed because of her health.

Nazreen also spoke about problems she has had at work regarding disclosure and stigmatization because of her positive HIV status. In one section of her interview she discussed a confrontation she had at a previous job with the boss of the small factory where she was doing ironing work.

> I go to my boss because I must tell her the steam from this iron isn't good for me, for this virus. So I go to her—lunchtime when she was alone—and I told her, "Umm, listen here, I'm HIV." "So! What must I do?!" she told me. So I said, "No, I'm just telling you that I'm HIV—isn't there something else that you can give me? Because the steam is not good for me." So she said, "I think you must just take your bag as well. Because I don't have time for you people. You must attend clinic or doctor every month. You must be in your work. Your work is your work." That is what she told me. So I took my bag and I go, because I don't need that.

Both Elaine's and Nazreen's stories are about their disclosure to their employers, but the stories have two very different endings. The differences illustrate how disclosure does not always have similar results for all people. People are encouraged by health-care workers and activists to disclose their status, but doing so can be perceived as a sign of weakness or vulnerability or can lead to weakness or vulnerability. Some women, such as Elaine, may be able to turn this vulnerability into a source of power, but others, such as Nazreen, may not be able to do so. Although laws have been made to protect people living with HIV, they are not necessarily abided by, and employees who disclose their HIV status are at the mercy of their bosses' decisions to either adhere to the laws or challenge the employees about their rights.

Disclosure to Families

Just as disclosures at work do not always have the same outcomes, disclosures to family members can also go either way. Although none of the open-ended interview questions we asked mentioned the word "family," the questions about disclosure elicited long discussions about the women's relationships with their families. The women described their struggles with their children and choosing to disclose or not disclose to them. They also expressed the need to disclose to their own mothers and spoke of the problems they faced in doing so. Some of this talk of children and mothers may be a product of gender identity, as the women may have felt that speaking about their children and mothers as central aspects of their lives was expected of them as good mothers and good daughters. The spontaneous discussion of family bonds and responsibilities, however, may also be due to the intense pressure they experience to disclose to people who are close to them as well as the strength of their feelings about the risk they would take in disclosing to their most intimate companions—their mothers and children.

Priscilla is one woman who spoke about disclosure—in particular, disclosure to her family. At the time of her interview, Priscilla had known of her HIV status for two years. Almost everyone in the support group talked about the huge initial blow of being diagnosed with HIV, but most group members who had known of their status for a year or more had somewhat come to terms with their HIV status. This was not the case for Priscilla. She had remained extremely upset and was emotionally run-down. She often cried during and after support group meetings. As a result, her counselors and support group facilitators repeatedly encouraged her to disclose her health condition to her family members. They had identified nondisclosure to her mother and daughter as her primary source of anxiety and believed that keeping this secret was both causing her great stress and isolating her from her best resource for social support.

> Sister ["sister" is the term used to address nurses in South Africa] Aisha, she told me I must disclose. She know it's not easy for me, but, umm, she know she is not the one with the virus, but I must just try to disclose. And if I don't have the courage to disclose, then I must just contact her or Nazeem [Sister Aisha's husband and the facilitator of the support group], and they will do the talking and they will exactly tell my people, my family, whatever . . . But, Anna, I'm not ready yet.

We asked Priscilla why she is not yet ready to disclose and she explained what she believed would happen upon her disclosure.

> I don't know if my mom is gonna accept me as her child. My mother's an alcoholic. I'm scared to tell my daughter. Really I'm very scared to tell her and my mother. . . . But I really want my mom, but I'm also scared, because right now she is standing in the public, telling the people who I am and what I am.

Priscilla describes her feelings about disclosure as being "scared" and seems torn about what to do. On the one hand, she feels pressure from the health-care and activist communities and the media to disclose her condition. On the other hand, she anticipates a stigmatizing response from her family members and from others in her community who may eventually find out, because she does not trust that her mother will keep her status private.

Denise is another woman we interviewed who also spoke about disclosing to her children. Like Pricilla, she had not yet told her family. Denise explained that she did not intend to disclose to anyone in the near future. She anticipated a bad reaction from her family and community and expected that the worst reaction would come from her children, in their early teens, who do not get along well with her.

ANNA: When . . . you said that no other people know now . . .

DENISE: No. Even my children doesn't know.

ANNA: Why have you decided not to tell your family?

DENISE: Because I'm still—HIV. You understand? If I got AIDS and all, umm . . . started to get my ARVs so I can tell them, but I'm not gonna tell my children, because *they* gonna tell the family—the family will tell them.

ANNA: Why don't you want them to know?

DENISE: Because they are rude. They stay with me and they are rude to me.

ANNA: The children? Your own children are rude?

DENISE: Yes.

ANNA: What do you mean they're rude?

DENISE: They don't respect me. They don't . . .

ANNA: If they found out . . . if your family told your children, how . . . what would they say to you—your children?

DENISE: Umm . . . I don't know what they gonna say, but the thing is I know they are rude. Like now, you know, I've got problems, but they always want to talk about their things in the group [other members of the support group], but I can't. Because every time when I want to talk, my eyes . . . they too full with tears, so I can't . . . [crying] . . .

ANNA: You feel sad when you talk about it.

DENISE: So I don't talk about it. I will tell. I will make time to talk and so I can feel better.

In the excerpt above, Denise tells us of the deep pain she feels in contemplating her dilemma of whether to disclose to her daughter or not. She is fearful and sad to even think about disclosing and what might happen if it does not go well. Denise, as well as several of the other women, has mixed feelings about the safety and effects of disclosure in her family life. In some ways she feels that disclosure might bring her some relief. At the end of this excerpt, for example, she says she will "make time to talk and so I can feel better." Here she is drawing on the discourse that she has heard in her support group, the media, and probably from health-care professionals she has encountered that disclosure leads to peace of mind, and she may fear that her pain stems from her reluctance to disclose. In the meantime, however, her fear of disclosure coupled with the pressure to disclose intensifies her feelings of anxiety and sadness.

The description of the risks and apprehension of disclosure we heard in Denise's discussion, and in our conversations with other women, suggests that perhaps people should not be encouraged to disclose their status if it causes such high levels of anxiety leading up to the disclosure. Disclosure is promoted as a way to increase social support for people living with HIV and as a way of relieving the stress of keeping secret such a difficult and important factor in their lives. But Denise and Pricilla explain to us that they know disclosure is deemed necessary by authority figures and that they are aware of the potential value of disclosing, but after careful consideration, in light of their own specific situations, they have come to the conclusion that it may not always be the best choice.

They are constantly reminded of this dilemma, because while there is great stress in keeping their HIV status a secret, they realize that disclosure has been successful in relieving stress for some of the other women in their support group. Elaine was one such woman. In response to a question about why she decided to get an HIV test, Elaine spoke with us about her disclosure, specifically to her children. She explained that once she decided to attend support group meetings and disclosed there, she began to reveal her status at home.

> Then I made myself strong and go to [the support group], and I get there and it's two years that I'm now with Nazeem [the support group leader] now. And I go there and I introduce myself 'cause they [the clinic where Elaine tested positive] gave me the address and they told me I must go there. And I introduced myself to them, and from that time on, I'm brave. I can talk . . . even afterwards I told my children I'm HIV positive and that I was okay, but I was crying. I couldn't tell them what's happening—what's wrong with me. Then I told my children, but my one daughter she was so crying. The other one just said, "Okay. It's fine, but we must all keep it confidential—we mustn't tell other people." And then my one daughter she was crying and crying.

Elaine speaks of the strength she gained in her support group disclosures and how this may have facilitated subsequent disclosures to her children. In fact, she claims to feel that a great burden was lifted once that disclosure took place. In response to a question in her interview about what her greatest worry is since finding out she is living with HIV, Elaine said, "I think I'm not anymore worried. I'm not anymore worried. Because the first thing that worried me was the children—how I'm gonna tell my children. Since I told them, I'm not worried anymore."

Linda, another participant who discussed disclosure with a positive outcome, at least in part, is the one person in the support group who described herself as living a relatively stress-free life. She spoke of having come to terms with her status and having supportive employers. Linda also told us that she quickly planned and executed a successful disclosure to her own children and other children in her family, and this proved to be an immensely positive decision. In this portion of the interview Linda tells the story of when she disclosed to all of the children.

> And my sister's children, because they're going together—they staying together. We just collected them. Then we sit down. It was Christmas Eve in the morning. Then they just sit on the floor. We closed the door, me and my sister. Then I asked them about what do they know about HIV. Each and every one saying anything that they know . . . "Yeah, HIV people can die . . ." Others said, "No, they can live longer . . ." You know . . . others say—they talking about a support group. We didn't know that they knew so much. I was so [impressed] . . .
>
> Then I told them, "Okay if somebody in this family is HIV—HIV positive—how are you going to react?" So the other ones said, "That person, whoever he is, we must support him—show them that we love him. Because at school they teach us that, and even if your friend is HIV positive, he's still your friend. And we can't get infected by chatting, hugging, sharing food—all those things. So there's nothing wrong with that . . ."
>
> So I think okay. Even those ones they just said, "HIV person he just die— he going to die," I can see—I did see that okay, they also now understand what is going on. Then I tell them . . . [crying] they all stood up and hugged me!

Linda maintains that she experienced a successful disclosure, which so far has benefited her. Nevertheless, she also spoke about a problem that remains: her struggle with the decision of disclosing to her elderly mother. In her comments she explained that while disclosure may be beneficial to the person living with HIV, we must also be mindful of the needs of other people who have other, equally difficult problems that might be exacerbated by finding out that someone they love is living with HIV.

> My mother doesn't know yet. She's old so when I think about her . . . because in 2004 my brother passed away. There were three of us. It was my brother and me and Mary [Linda's sister]. So my brother passed away, so it was difficult for my mom. So sometimes I think I can't tell her . . . I . . . maybe she will be devastated. Because, you know, elder people they believe in that it's better them to pass away and leave us behind, because if we passed away, who's gonna bury them? They believe in that, you know. So we discussed with my sister. My sister say, "Just keep it that way."

In addition, when we asked Linda about what things need to be improved or changed to better help women living with the virus, she spoke of the need to educate families of women living with HIV.

> It's a long way to go . . . because even in the families—especially in the families . . . So you can be supported by other people, but the important support is from the family. If the family doesn't support you, those people—they can't do anything. They can help you with things that they can help, but as a woman, if you

got children, you see? We think that, ooh . . . if someday my days have come—
what about my children? Because the important person who can look after
your children is your family. So if the family is not supporting you, where are
you going to leave the children? Where? It's . . . it's difficult. So if maybe people
can get more knowledge—especially the family. Because other people like us,
like in the support group—we support each other. We don't care—we just love
each other, and we share what we have, but the families . . . it's difficult. It's the
most important support.

Interestingly, Linda suggests that fear of disclosure to family is not based on
potential stigma; rather, it is a practical fear of losing support. Not only is she
concerned about support for her and her children now, but she is also concerned
about being able to call on family to help her with her children and arranging
her life so that her children can survive when she is gone. Linda's assessment is
also noteworthy because she suggests that sources outside of her family should
be called upon to develop educational programs for families of people living with
HIV. In this way she is challenging policy makers and health-care providers to
supplement or to even replace what has been assumed to be the burden and responsibility of HIV-positive people and their families.

Linda agrees fundamentally with the tenets of the dominant disclosure discourse and points out a more practical benefit of disclosure for women in particular: the issue of who will help with her children when she is sick or dying.
However, again Linda sees some of her personal issues surrounding disclosure as
an exception to the rule.

If the family maybe can be taught and understand. Except that like me—my
mother . . . I know maybe she can't understand, but my mother she's got . . .
she's eating the treatment of high blood pressure. Maybe she can understand,
but back of her mind, sometimes she would think, "Oh! . . . which means . . ."
Because everyone knew this rumor without understanding that it's not like
that. Everyone knows that if someone's HIV positive, she's gonna die—and it's
not like that! So she will feel like, "Okay, I heard people do that . . . now my
child!" You see? They don't understand, especially elder people—they don't
understand.

Elvyra is another participant in our study who attends the support group,
works as a peer counselor, and stresses the importance of HIV disclosure in sessions with her clients. She disclosed her own HIV status to her family over fifteen years ago, but unlike Linda's and Elaine's families, Elvyra's reacted negatively.
Her mother insisted she use separate eating utensils and was concerned about her
toothbrush being near the rest of the family's toothbrushes. Only recently has
Elvyra's youngest sister approached her and asked Elvyra to forgive her for years
of estrangement. Despite the long-term negative effects of her disclosure, Elvyra
emphasized the importance of disclosure to the family.

ELVYRA: If you got a good counselor and your family's support—you get a family that supports you, then nothing will go wrong.

ANNA: Do you think the counselors are good?

ELVYRA: Some counselors are very good. They very good.

ANNA: Is that person the most important support in the whole process?

ELVYRA: Sometimes it is your family. If you got a family that supports you all the way, then you feel very good. If you've got no family that supports you in this, then you will have problems all the time.

ANNA: What do you tell people if you were counseling and they said, "I can't tell my family," or "My family hates me now." What do you tell them?

ELVYRA: I will tell them just fast and pray. Your family will come to you. Someday all the other—your family will come. Because now the other . . . you know who's coming to visit me and phoning me now and then? My baby sister. So my friends said, "[gasp] Wow! What?" So no. So I said to my friend, "Just pray. Pray every day and ask God just to forgive her [Elvyra's sister] for what she told the other people, and she will come right one day."

The medical discourse tells people living with HIV that they must disclose their status at least to those whom they are closest to. This is undoubtedly sound advice for many, but the women in our study explained that while disclosure is difficult, it may also sometimes be dangerous, especially disclosing to our closest family members. The women presented equally sound reasons not to disclose—for example, if the people closest to them cannot handle the news, or if the women might lose essential practical support in their already precarious situation. In addition to facing further stigmatization and rejection, they risk losing necessary everyday support for themselves and their children. They may also lose future care for their children after they have died, and they may harm those closest to them who are not living with HIV but who face their own economic, social, and health problems.

Disclosure to Strangers

It was apparent that disclosure is a complicated decision to make, and many times it is simply too risky. The risk is not just one of stigmatization. Nearly all of the women we interviewed identified the loss of social and material support—jobs, family support for children, a house to live in—as the risk they believe they are taking with disclosure. However, it is interesting that some of the women have enthusiastically disclosed to quite a few people who are relative strangers—for example, coworkers or new people in the support group—if not complete strangers they meet on the street. It is perhaps not surprising that they are less afraid of hostility from strangers than the removal of material and emotional support by family members. A good example of this kind of random disclosure is evident in Elaine's words when she spoke about being on a roll in terms of disclosures. She told us the story of one of the many times she has revealed her HIV status to a relative stranger.

> Or if I'm drunk, I walk in the street, I tell this person . . . "*Jy!* [Afrikaans for 'Hey, you'], you know what? I'm HIV positive. Leave me alone." There was one guy—he's a church-goer. He talked to me about God. I said, "No, I don't want to listen about God." I was *lekker* [Afrikaans for good and] drunk that night. I went home. I said, "I'm HIV positive." He came to me the next day or the next week—came to ask me if I want to go with him to church. I said, "No, I don't want to go with you to church." He asked me, "Do you know what you told me yesterday?" I said, "Yes, I know what I told you! But don't come and pity me because I'm HIV positive."

In disclosures to strangers, Elaine is fulfilling the need to disclose, just as many other people living with HIV are pressured to do. This type of disclosure might be considered safer than a disclosure to a family member, because there is less to lose. Elaine spoke of another occasion, in which she disclosed to a coworker with whom she was not very close.

> Yes, and that other lady at work also said to me I'm very strong. She said to me, "You very strong woman. Because why? Other people don't want to talk about their status. They don't want to tell nothing." I said, "No, if you talk, then you can make yourself better." If you keep yourself in like Priscilla—Priscilla don't want to talk. That's why Priscilla is always crying and crying and crying, because she don't want to talk. You must talk. If you talk, you talk the sickness away from you . . . but if you sit and cry . . .

In this instance Elaine may have taken a great risk in disclosing to a coworker; nevertheless, her colleague reacted positively to the disclosure. In the above excerpt, Elaine tells how "talking" about one's status "can make you feel better" and points to Priscilla's pain being a direct result of her reluctance to speak about her status.

Contrary to Elaine's belief, however, Priscilla has disclosed to relative strangers as well. She told us about the disclosures she has made to the teachers and principal at the school her children attend.

> PRISCILLA: I go to my two boys' school. I go tell the principal—I think they must know if anything . . . maybe like the two boys is at home for more than a month, then they must think, "But that boy's mommy is sick." So you see? I just go to the principal and to my eldest son, Ryan, and I go to his teacher.
>
> ANNA: How did they react?
>
> PRISCILLA: The principal did call the two teachers to the office, and so they prayed for me. Yes, and, umm, that's all. So I go to my daughter's high

school, go see her teacher. So the teacher come to the office and I told her about it. Maybe if there's anything that if Lizle [Priscilla's daughter] is more than a month out of school, then they must just think, "Maybe Lizle's mommy is sick." But she said she will contact me—she will come and make a turn by there [pay a visit to Priscilla's home]. That's the only people that know—my partner and my eldest daughter's teacher and my two boys and the principal and teachers.

Priscilla relates the practical reasons for these disclosures, but these are not the only relative strangers to whom she has disclosed. Priscilla participates in public disclosures held at churches in various neighborhoods in Cape Town. She described what a relief these church disclosures are and how good it feels when a whole room of people is praying for her. In addition, Priscilla talked at length about her time collecting donations at a supermarket, where her status was made public with a sign above her table reading "Support People Living With HIV/AIDS." Here she talks about how she reacted to shoppers who inquired about her status.

You know, so . . . there was a part of me I didn't like the idea, but you know . . . so time just go and come by, so I just said, no, if they come and ask me again, then I'm gonna be just honest. Because I don't know the place—I don't know the people. So kids, children came to me.

Here Priscilla claims to have empowered herself by disclosing to strangers, but only because she is not from the area and does not know the people there.

These random or spur-of-the-moment disclosures are interesting because Elaine and Priscilla, like many other women living with the virus, do not consider themselves as "out" in regard to their status. For example, Elaine, who has been able to disclose to complete strangers and distant coworkers, also talked about her need for privacy in the matter.

There was another lady also, I think from work . . . "I heard you got AIDS." "Oh," I said, "Who told you so?" "No, I heard the people say you've got AIDS." I said, "If I've got AIDS, it's got nothing to do with nobody." I said, "The people likes to talk a lot of things." That's why since I got this I haven't got friends anymore, because all the friends that I had are gone. And if I told them I'm HIV positive, then the whole world will know that I'm HIV positive.

In the above excerpt, Elaine states that, possibly because some people to whom she has disclosed have not kept the information confidential, she has lost friends. Because social support is so scarce, her loss of friends may have been a high price to pay for having disclosed as the dominant discourses say people should.

Priscilla, who has also publicly disclosed, has expressed her frustration with not being able to disclose to the people closest to her. Here she explains what happens each time she visits her doctor.

Because when I go to my doctor, it's every month just cry, cry, cry, cry. I don't know . . . Every time when I sit home, I'm fine. But every time it's my checkup for my doctor, then I just cry and cry . . . He said it's great to cry. He said I must talk, and if I want to cry, then I must cry—I will feel better. And it's true. When I cry, then I feel better. And when I'm talking and . . . I feel better . . . Then he asks me, "What is it, Priscilla? What's wrong?" Then I tell him, "I still live with this secret in me for two whole years. I don't know how to disclose. I'm scared to disclose." So he told me, "If you are scared, just leave it. Maybe you will tell your family or your parents or what-what . . . just leave it." But every time, Anna, when I go and see the doctor, then just tears. I don't know why.

Priscilla explains here how her doctor encourages her to talk and cry as a way to feel better. Ironically, she says, upon hearing her pain and frustration regarding disclosure, this same doctor says that if she is scared to disclose, then she should "just leave it." On one hand the dominant discourses pressure people to disclose, but in this example we can see that even some members of the medical community believe that disclosure is complicated and anxiety-provoking and, especially, that for some people the risks might outweigh the benefits.

Structural and Personal Challenges in the Decision to Disclose

Even though stigma is both a perceived and real barrier to disclosure, Priscilla and Elaine have been able to disclose in certain situations with mixed results. The contradiction is that they want to and do disclose to relative strangers, but at the same time they claim to be unable to disclose to at least some of those who are closest to them, because they physically need those people to stay close. Ironically, the reason the medical community believes people living with HIV should disclose to their families (because their families are their main source of practical support) is the same reason it is such a risk to take in case it fails. If their families or employers reject them, they are abandoned without the material support necessary to survive; equally devastating, after they die, their children will be without material support from those who have abandoned them.

Discourses of disclosure are important as they relate to HIV and medical treatment and psychosocial support (Klitzman et al., 2004). Practically speaking, disclosure is legally required for people who are living with the virus and wish to obtain government and community resources (Castle, 2004), specifically, ARV treatment. In fact, the Antiretroviral Treatment Protocol for the Western Cape (Provincial Administration Western Cape, 2004) requires a person to disclose to "at least one friend or family member or have joined a support group" (p. 4). The premise of this policy rests on the notion in the medical community in South Africa, and in many other parts of the world, that disclosure facilitates psychosocial support, which has a buffering effect against HIV stigma (Friedland, Renwick & McColl, 1996). The medical community also asserts that disclosure, to partners in particular, offers a psychological release that is beneficial to psychological health and, in turn, beneficial to physical health (Derlega, Winstead, Greene, Serovich & Elwood, 2002). This notion of disclosure as a type of catharsis is also reflected in the data obtained from our own study as well as in Squire's (2007) research involving HIV-positive people in South Africa.

In addition to the material, emotional, and social support that may be gained upon disclosure, the South African media and activist communities like the CADRE (Centre for AIDS Research and Evaluation), the TAC (Treatment Action Campaign), and the HSRC (Human Sciences Research Council) have created and propagated a counter discourse calling for social change in the realm of HIV stigma. It is the agenda of these agencies to advocate HIV disclosure as a way of restructuring society such that stigma becomes an impossibility. It is the view of many activists that by inducing a sort of mass disclosure of all persons living with the virus, HIV stigma could be abolished.

Many of the women we interviewed have such a strong anticipation of stigma and rejection that they cannot bring themselves to disclose. This fear to disclose—in South Africa in particular—may have to do with discourses of fear set forth by the media in their perhaps overreporting of events involving HIV-related violence and discrimination (Squire, 2007). Nevertheless, stigma is omnipresent, it is layered and multidimensional (Fife & Wright, 2000), and the fear of stigma upon disclosure may be due to numerous factors. One factor we noted in our study is the commonly voiced problem of not knowing how to disclose. The women in the support group shared their fears in group meetings. They explained that a great part of their fear comes from not knowing how to create the setting for disclosure and not knowing how to predict if the friend or family member will react negatively. This idea also encapsulates the struggle they have with disclosing to their mothers and children in particular. The medical and activist establishment may be right in their advocacy of disclosure, but within their messages is the assumption that orchestrating successful disclosures is a skill that most people inherently have. It most certainly is not. In addition, these messages fail to take into account that each disclosure has its own unique set of circumstances, including barriers, fears, and consequences, that women in particular must anticipate.

The problem with lack of instruction on how to disclose was illustrated when women in the support group expressed their need to "predict the future." As with the women in studies conducted by Doyal and Anderson (2006) as well as by Kimberly and her colleagues (1995), disclosing to elderly mothers was a source of great anxiety. There was an expressed fear that the disclosure may kill their mothers, who may be living with their own social or health problems. The related fear of disclosing to children is also a complex one. The women we interviewed grappled with the dilemma of wanting to disclose their status to their children and their fear of the subsequent stigmatization of their children, who may or may not also be HIV positive. This finding is supported by similar findings in the Schrimshaw and Siegel (2002) study of American women living with HIV.

As described in this chapter, for the women in our study, making the decision to disclose their HIV status has been confusing and at times impossible. The medical and psychological establishments as well as the HIV activist community are putting pressure on them to disclose in order to gain social, material, and medical resources; make changes in the way society sees people living with HIV; and to serve as a catharsis. No matter how great the gains may be, however, disclosing is easier said than done. The women in our study point out that it is not always possible to disclose publicly, especially if there are no support systems in place to facilitate successful disclosures and assist with the difficulty of predicting the reactions of the loved ones to whom they may choose to disclose. And perhaps most important is that there are few support systems in place to replace the material resources families provide that might be jeopardized if the disclosure does not go well.

Even while the professional community advocates disclosure, it offers little to compensate women if a disclosure results in rejection by the extended family on which she depends for support. Unless communities and governments can come up with a social safety net that extends beyond family boundaries, disclosure is a huge gamble and a risk that is cruel to demand of people living with HIV. The intense discussion of the dilemma of disclosure among the women in this study and the decision by so many of them not to disclose points to the need to move beyond seeing HIV as something that can be addressed one person at a time. Rather it shows us how much we need to do to change the broader social context in order to truly develop effective and humane ways of tackling HIV.

Furthermore, in our reflection on these issues we need to be ever mindful of the effects of gender. Disclosure is difficult for everyone, but it is especially difficult for women because of their family responsibilities. For example, many of them are afraid their children will be stigmatized if their mother's HIV status is revealed. They also fear the emotional reaction of their children, because many children are especially close to their mothers. In addition, their care responsibilities for other family members, such as their own mothers, also confounds their deliberations about disclosure. Finally, disclosure is gendered and more difficult for women because of their economic vulnerability.

6 Staking a Claim as Normal through Work and Relationships with Men

STIGMATIZATION APPEARS TO be a major barrier for women to overcome in order to disclose their HIV status. While stigmatization is a critical factor for everyone living with HIV, the force of stigmatization may be intensified in specific ways for women, since they must make their way through the multiple layers of challenges of particularly gendered forms of HIV stigmatization. Gendered HIV stigma may be internalized, causing psychological pain, or it may manifest itself in more concrete ways, such as preventing women from working or going to school and thus making them feel they are not valued members of society and unable to realize their full potential as human beings. Nevertheless, women find ways of shielding or "disguising" themselves from the full force of gendered HIV stigma and othering that takes place in their lives. One way women respond is to find ways to normalize themselves. Discourses about men and about work emerged in our interviews as normalizing processes to counter stigma.

Working Is Normal

Work is an important part of most people's lives—we earn money through work so that we can pay our expenses. Some people earn enough money through work to live relatively easy lives, but most people in the world earn very little money and must work for wages just to scrape by. For the women we interviewed, work is important for survival, but it also represents something more and is meaningful on several different levels.

The following fund-raising story that Priscilla told us in her interview illustrates the special importance of work. The support group in which she participates receives funding from the government, but the demand for services and support exceeds the funding. In order for this support group (and groups like it in the Western Cape) to sustain services to members, fund-raising events are held. A common fund-raising strategy is to set up tables in shopping malls and supermarkets and request donations or sell small items such as red ribbons or crafts that the group members have made. Priscilla explained how she was asked by the facilitator of her HIV support group to sit alone with her baby daughter at a fund-raising table in a local supermarket to collect money for the organization. Above the table a banner was hung with the name of the support group and a sign reading "Support People Living with HIV/AIDS" painted in bold letters.

> Now I was sitting there and the people is looking at me and looking at my baby, you know? I can see they feel ashamed for me. And, umm, "What's your name? . . . Are you HIV?" the people come and ask me. "Is this baby also HIV? . . . Is this your baby? Because it's a very beautiful baby . . . Are you looking after this baby? . . . Is this infant HIV?"

A situation like this, where a sign above her head announced her HIV status, could have been distressing and a potential source of enormous stigma or othering for Priscilla. The banner served to draw a distinct line between someone living with HIV and the "normal" customers at the supermarket. However, Priscilla described how as the days went by she began to adjust to sitting under the banner.

Part of the reason she became more comfortable had to do with the clothing and monetary donations she was receiving, specifically for herself and her daughter. But she also talked about something that went beyond receiving donations. Priscilla explained how much she began to look forward to waking up in the morning to go to work at the fund-raising table simply because it was work. These positive feelings were quite significant for Priscilla, especially because she had to ready herself and her infant daughter in the morning with no electricity or running water, and many times no food for herself or her child. Just like the other employees in the store, she had to arrive at a particular time on a regular schedule, and her assignment was to work as a community educator, responding to the inquiries of the shoppers who stopped by her table. In return, she received monetary donations for both herself and the support group. This job stigmatized Priscilla because of the disclosure of her HIV status, but she feels that the fact that it was work and that it resulted in material benefits for her and her child allowed her to be a normal and respectable member of the community.

> And I really miss that shop. I really miss that supervisor, especially two or three ladies who's also working on the tills. But I was feeling better. And every night then they come and pick me up, and I have something new that the people bought my baby, you know, in the shop. I was really enjoying myself, and, you know, Anna, when they come in the morning—come and pick me up, then I was . . . I was so glad. "Oh, I'm going to work." I didn't put in my mind that I'm going to sit there the whole day feeling shy.

Priscilla underscores how important it is to her to have a way to provide for her child in ways that were previously unavailable to her because of limited job opportunities due to race and gender disparities in the labor market, discrimination against people living with HIV, and the high rates of unemployment in South Africa in general. In addition to the modest financial benefit, she seems to be eager to be involved in a work activity that could possibly allow her to feel like there is a purpose in her waking up each morning. Those of us who have been unemployed for a period of time can relate to what Priscilla is describing here. When we are not working, not only are we under pressure because we do not have the money we need, but we are also at loose ends in other ways. Being able to "go to work" gives our lives structure and often a sense of value and feelings of satisfaction.

Priscilla is saying that by working she becomes a worthy person, she can provide a service for the community, she can make money, and she deserves to be seen as a valuable human being. It appears that Priscilla does not call upon her humanity to make this case to herself or others. Instead, she calls upon her ability to work and her success at working to earn some material things as an indication of her human value to herself, her child, and to everyone around her. Priscilla's description of her feelings is ironic. On one hand, she explains that it makes her feel good and that it brings her happiness to be able to work. On the other hand, however, she points to a power structure that sees little value in her or her child, except if she can be "productive" and earn her keep.

Linda, another support group member, also told us about work and how she first learned about her HIV status. She is employed as a domestic worker in the home of a wealthy family consisting of a wife, husband, and a young son, for whom Linda cares during the day. Her employers have known about her status from the beginning, because the wife was with Linda in the doctor's office when her positive HIV test result was revealed. At one point after Linda's diagnosis and commencement of her ARV treatment, her employers asked her if she needed to quit her job and go back to another large South African city where Linda's family resides.

> I was so . . . I did really cry very hard. Because they asked me now that I'm sick—now that I'm HIV . . . blah, blah, blah . . . I was already taking ARVs, so what must I do? Or maybe I want to go back home and stay at home not working . . . I just panicked. I said this means they are chasing me away. I just cried.

The thought of not working causes Linda psychological distress as she describes how "not working" elicited panic in the excerpt above. Losing her job has important economic implications, of course, but her anguish also suggests that losing her job will mean cutting important social and emotional ties as her employer "chases her away."

She and her employers eventually resolved this problem and Linda retained her job. She says she is now in a good position with regard to her job stability, and in our interview she was actually able to laugh at how worried she was at the time as she went on to explain her fear of leaving or being fired from her job.

> LINDA: You know what, if I go back home . . . I think I'm gonna die quickly [laughing].
> ANNA: Oh no!

LINDA: Yes [laughing]! Because, you know, your children knows that you are working. Okay, you come back home, now my children know I'm sick, and you scared to tell your children what sickness you have. And also then if they don't understand—when they look at you they will think that any time you gonna die.

Linda expresses the notion of work and death as polar opposites. She says that being unemployed is like dying and speaks of her dread of thinking about how her children will experience her death. Once again the relationship between her humanity and her ability to work seem to be contradictory. She says that continuing to work signifies to herself that she is not all that ill. When she says that leaving her job may cause her to "die quickly," she is saying that without work she would not be a productive, contributing, and living member of the community. Yet it also expresses the power relationship that places her in the position of having to "earn her keep" or go off and die.

The following excerpt from our interview with Elaine illustrates this same contradiction. Elaine reiterates how important it is to her that her work abilities in a large factory be recognized despite problems that may arise because of her illness.

I told the people at work also. . . . I said to them, "I don't want pity. I don't want people to pity me. I just want people to be with me as they are—as I am . . . they used to be with me—just be with me as you are—as you used to be. Don't pity me. Because why? When you pity me, then I'm gonna think, Oh! The people is pitying me." And then they told me at work, "You must work like any other person . . . like any other person . . . you must work like any other person. And we gonna treat you like any other person. We not gonna treat you like you are a sick person."

Elaine repeatedly indicates that she wants to "work like any other person," despite her HIV status. Her words here tell us that, for her, working signifies being normal.

As the above excerpts illustrate, the subject of work surfaced in our conversations in many forms. Sometimes work was mentioned as a problem that causes psychological stress. Work also emerged as part of the discussion of the economic challenges a woman faces. Most interestingly, work was described as an indication of normalcy; a woman who wishes to be a "regular working person" despite the virus in her body might find that work makes her normal. In all of these three examples in which the discussion of work took place, the link between work and normalcy can be traced back to complex power and sociopolitical factors—some of which are unique to South Africa.

The context of the women's comments and the particular way in which South African history as well as the current political and economic landscape relate to what the women said about work are discussed at the end of this chapter. But first let us look at a second way that women stake a claim to normalcy and acceptability, this time through their relationships with men. Talk of relationships and sex with men as a device for appearing to be normal despite harboring the abnormality of living with HIV was a noticeable pattern in many of the women's narratives.

Having a Man Is Normal

Elvyra is married to a man who refuses to be tested for HIV and who also refuses to wear condoms. Although throughout our interview Elvyra spoke at length and at many times about her husband's refusal to use condoms, she was surprisingly uncritical of his refusal and might truly be unconcerned with this issue. More likely, however, is that what seems to be her acceptance of his nonuse of condoms may instead be related to another discourse surrounding gender power structures. In theory a woman can easily ask a man, even a husband, to wear a condom, but in practice this request becomes complicated. In reality, wives who request condom use may become suspect by their husbands, because married couples are not "supposed" to use condoms (One in Nine, 2012). Some women fear or actually experience violence at the hands of their partner as a result of attempting to use condoms. In fact, while our study took place, we were also involved in distributing condoms in local nightclubs in the Cape Town area. This gendered stigma against condoms became clear as several men intervened when their partners or girlfriends were handed condoms. More than a few men explained that only women doing sex work needed to be given condoms. Some men took the condoms out of the hands of their partner or girlfriend and gave them back to us, deeply offended. In many cases condom negotiation for women is simply unacceptable. Along with stigma and possible violence, scholars have also observed women's fear that the financial resources her husband is providing will be revoked if they ask their husbands to use condoms (Hoosen & Collins, 2004; Petros, Airhihenbuwa, Simbayi, Ramlagan & Brown, 2006).

In Elvyra's case, she is the breadwinner in her household. Her husband is not providing any financial support. The reason for the nonuse of condoms in her situation, therefore, may be due to her wish to have what she perceives as a normal sexual relationship with her husband. In a discussion about her family's reaction to her status, she moved from discussing her family's rejection to talking about a new person who has entered her life.

> And I've got this man in my life now . . . I . . . we were married thirty years ago, but he was in jail all the years. . . . So two years ago we met each other again and we got married last year. Next month we married a year—March we married a year . . . So I went to go visit him in jail, so he must have heard by my family that, "Elvyra is sick." So I said to him, "Yeah, I am sick." So he said,

okay, it's his choice and he don't want to lose me again. So we got married and we living together now. And so I said to him, "Anyway, I don't want you also to get sick, because then we both is gonna get sick. We can't look after each other. Either you must use a condom . . ." So he said, no, he's not gonna use a condom . . . he's not gonna use a condom. So we having unprotected sex.

Elvyra has attempted to use condoms, and she explains how her husband has refused, but something that is lost in the transcription of her interview is how she conveyed this story to us. Elvyra is very proud when she speaks about her husband and their marriage, even when she explains this failed attempt at condom negotiation. The positive way in which she told us this story implies that she would like to be seen as having been a part of the decision to not use condoms or that she fully supports her husband's refusal. In addition, she appears to be proud of her married status and that she and her husband are having what she perceives as a normal sex life—in other words, no condoms. It is important to note that Elvyra works as a peer counselor for people living with HIV. One of her duties is to describe the importance of the use of condoms in sexual relationships and to offer advice to women on how to protect their health through condom negotiation. When we take this into consideration, it becomes clear how powerful this gendered discourse around how married people should have sex and what role women play in the negotiation of their sex life really is.

Also of note in this excerpt is Elvyra's choice to reunite with a man to whom she was previously married and divorced before her subsequent marriage, in which she became infected with HIV. It is possible that the man she is now married to may represent her life as it once was—she has taken back this man from her past, possibly because he symbolizes her life when it was still normal.

Talk of not using condoms as part of being normal arose again in our interview with Rosalind, who is also a volunteer peer counselor for couples who have recently tested positive for HIV. She spoke about what she tells her own clients in counseling sessions.

And it's not the end of the world if you're positive. Yes, I tell them. I tell the couple, "It's not the end of the world. If you want to use a condom, you can use a condom, but don't go to other partners. Sleep with each other. Stay with each other if you don't want to use a condom."

Rosalind is suggesting that monogamy negates the necessity for condoms to be used by couples who are HIV positive. Her advice to these couples expresses her beliefs about what it means to be in a normal partnership or marriage.

Being normal as a function of having a relationship with a man was seen again when Elaine spoke about a confrontation with a woman who was rudely commenting on Elaine's thin body.

> The other day, the other woman said to me, "Oh, you so thin! Your boyfriend is too long—so tall!" . . . She said, "I'm 57 and I don't even have a boyfriend." I said, "That's nothing to do with me. That's your problem. I can't help if I've got a boyfriend who can help look after me. And you don't have one. That's your problem." "But you so thin and I'm so *lekker* fat and I . . ." I said, "That's nothing to do with me! That's nothing to do with me."

What Elaine is saying here is despite the fact that she's visibly living with HIV, she can still attract men and maintain a relationship. Elaine's conversation with this woman is significant because Elaine has been stigmatized and publicly humiliated by the people in her neighborhood. She lives in public housing, where many people reside in close proximity and where there are tight networks of friends and family, which, she says, means little privacy when it comes to her HIV status.

She frequently mentioned her boyfriend during the interview in such a way that suggests she is proud that he is part of her life and that although he is not perfect, he brings a sense of normalcy to it. She continues to emphasize the seriousness of her partnership with her boyfriend in this discussion of the possibility of marriage.

> He said to me he wants . . . I asked him, "Now, why do you want to marry me?" "No, Elaine, I know we are together—we can stay together." "And okay, I'm just waiting for that time to come. I'm not going to give you no . . ." But I said to him, "If you want to get married, we must get married on your birthday." And I told him, you know what—the 27th! I was married also on the 27th that time. Now, his birthday is also on the 27th of June. Now, I said to him, "Imagine now I'm going to get married again on the 27th of June!" He said to me, "No, but it's fine! It's on my birthday." I said, "Yes, but that time I didn't know your name. I didn't know you. But now you—the 27th of June." But I don't know if we are gonna get married. But he said to me, "I want to marry you, but you mustn't tell anybody now at this moment. I want to make it a surprise. Don't even tell the children. I want to make it a surprise." I said, "Okay."

Elaine is excited when she repeatedly describes her hopes of marriage and "getting married." Like Elvyra, Elaine's hope of a marriage may represent a passport back into the normal world. She believes that the trauma of a positive HIV status can be turned around with a newly acquired status of "married."

Talking around Work and Relationships with Men in Context

The history of work as a discourse in the context of postapartheid South Africa is complex and layered with different meanings for different people. Apartheid, a political and judicial system constructed by the white South African government (described in chapter 2), was based on the imposed physical and social separation of people based on their constructed racial classification system (Salo,

2005). One of the ironies that resulted from these restrictions was that Coloured women living in the Western Cape had an advantage over Coloured men in the labor market. When it came to working, women were more likely than men to be able to find paid jobs and often became the primary breadwinners during apartheid (Boonzaier, 2001). This is quite different from black South Africans' experience. Black men were sometimes given passes to enter white areas to work, and in the Cape Town area they lived in men's hostels far away from the city center. Although some black women were permitted passes to enter Cape Town to work as domestic workers, they were usually completely barred from entering the Western Cape. Coloured people, especially Coloured women, however, were permitted to enter "whites only" areas to work.

In addition to the specific historical context of apartheid, work is also a reflection of a person's worth in most nations in the world. Capitalist economies do not place value on humans or grant them rights as a result of their humanity. Humans who do not own wealth are valued only in terms of how much work they can do in a given amount of time. Consequently, work is what most of us spend the majority of our time doing, and many people define themselves according to their ability to do a job. On one hand, this issue of defining oneself through one's ability to do work can be dehumanizing in that we are primarily a measure of our ability to enrich our employers. In contrast, work is also an important and potentially a joyful part of being a human. In a United Kingdom study of women from eleven African countries living with HIV, Doyal and Anderson (2006) found that the women expressed their desire to work as a way to put their lives back together and to contribute to society. These women also expressed the belief that working gives them freedom and greater control over their lives.

Another explanation for how the women we interviewed made work a focal point is given by Hoosen and Collins (2004) in their study on discourses of gender and HIV in KwaZulu-Natal, South Africa. The two researchers theorize that the people in their study may have repressed their threatening or traumatic thoughts about HIV because those thoughts hinder their psychological functioning. It is possible that the women we interviewed also chose to talk about work because conversing about something other than their health provides relief from talking about their positive HIV status and takes their minds off the constant, exhausting thoughts about living with the virus. In addition, talking about work allows them to emphasize other aspects of themselves and their lives. It permits them to present another piece of their identity, one that fits the criteria of "normal." Work is both a way to prove that one is alive and a contributing member of a community as well as something to discuss that is apart from one's HIV status. In our conversations with Pricilla, Linda, and Elaine, they did not avoid talking about HIV, but they emphasized their work lives. The women tied the two issues together, explaining that work allows them to see themselves as something more than being HIV positive. Through work they are contributing members of their families and communities and are therefore normal.

Many people see work as a defining characteristic of themselves or as a major part of their identity and an activity that signifies being normal. But besides work, other discourses or particular ideas that people speak about are related to the issue of appearing to be normal. In other places in our interviews, women talked about seeking acknowledgment for being activists in the fight against HIV. Paradoxically, or perhaps as an addition to their complex selves, they spoke of the need to be viewed by others as normal people. This is a discourse related to ideas that have emerged about poverty and women's health that indicates how women are blamed for their predicament. Blaming the victim deflects attention, especially critical attention, from more structural sources or from other sections of society that have failed to address social problems or have even caused the problems themselves, such as the government or the economy.

The dominant discourse of poverty—the "culture of poverty" model—is that women who are poor are somehow responsible for getting themselves into difficult situations because of poor choices and decisions they have made (Reid & Tom, 2006). Similarly, within this model, poor women's health problems are their own faults. As a result of this dominant discourse, women who fall outside the norm of "good decision makers" and who have become infected with HIV are not only deemed abnormal but also accused of being victims of their own bad behavior, bad values, and bad nature. The women we interviewed countered this stereotype by pointing out their successes, especially their successes in the labor market, as evidence of their value and normalcy.

The discourse of work emerged as a theme in our interviews because work is how many people measure their worth. The ability to work is viewed as valuable in capitalist societies, and it is seen as a type of status symbol in South Africa, a sign of one's humanity and value to others. The women we interviewed spoke about work being a way to show society that they are valuable and normal women. However, work is not the only vehicle by which women living with HIV are able to boost themselves back up from "being HIV" to "being normal." The women in our study also expressed a sense of normalcy in a life that is marginalized in many ways, including being HIV positive, by having a man partner or husband in their talk of boyfriends, husbands, monogamy, and marriage. Having a partner or husband is a symbol of status as well as a cry out to society, saying, "If this man values me, then so should you!"

"If this man values me, then so should you"

The perception that it is necessary to have a man partner to achieve acceptance and normality is related to another social construct: marriage or monogamous marriage-like relationships. Marriage has been described by Sibonile Ellece (2011) as "the building block of all societies, and is considered a safe haven for bringing up children and ensuring that they become balanced and productive citizens" (p. 43). It is an institution that is linked to respectability because it is closely associated with ideas of legitimized sexuality, provision of appropriate upbringing for children, and being a part of stable and moral activity (Marso, 2010). For many South Africans, those who are married or in marriage-like relationships can fulfill expectations of having children and "knit[ting] them[selves] into the networks of alliance in the township . . . ensur[ing] their long-term survival in their communities" (Salo, 2006, p. 8). In addition, marriage is perceived to provide a safe haven from HIV. South African research by Hoosen and Collins (2004), for example, found that the participants constructed marriage as a monogamous arrangement and a refuge from HIV. But for women (not to mention marginalized men), the positive beliefs and descriptions of marriage that are commonly held are not a reality. Marriage, at least the way it is defined in dominant ideology and most legal systems, is also recognized as a tool of oppression that works to maintain systems of gender inequality, gender injustice, and heteronormativity (Msibi, 2011). For example, in most nations marriage is defined as a relationship between one man and one woman. Marriage within this framework (which is a typical construction of marriage) immediately excludes relationships in same-sex couples and therefore upholds heteronormativity. Marriage in many legal systems and most dominant ideologies also include rules and regulations about heterosexual relationships. Women may be obligated to give up their names, their inheritance, their land, or their paycheck to their husbands, and they may be required to defer to their husbands in order to fulfill the criteria of being a properly married woman.

Furthermore, despite the common discourses around the safety and security that marriage is supposed to provide, for South Africans as well as in many other nations, marriage is actually an unsafe space in terms of exposure to HIV (UNAIDS/UNFPA/UNIFEM, 2004). Mlondi kaNdlondlo (2011) writes about South African women's construction of marriage, particularly his own mother's, and their subsequent vulnerability to HIV because of the stigma attached to leaving a marriage. For his mother's generation, "marriage acts as a form of currency: she is better than all the women who never married because no man wanted them" (p. 19). Even when women are aware that their husbands are HIV positive or are engaging in sex practices that may make them vulnerable to HIV, they are locked into marriage because of the equally problematic choice of leaving their husbands and then being forced to become misfits in a society that expects women to be married.

Furthermore, women locked into relationships in which their husbands may be likely to infect them with HIV have little power to control their sexual encounters by demanding that their husbands use condoms. Married women are often less likely than unmarried women to be able to protect themselves from HIV by using condoms. In their work in Zambia, for example, Chireshe and Chireshe (2011) found that because of their greater ability to negotiate condom use, unmarried women were more protected from HIV than women who were married.

For the women in our study, who are already living with HIV, marriage and marriage-like relationships become doubly important. The women we interviewed do indeed construct marriage and relationships with men as something positive and necessary, but they are also dealing with the sad irony that their marriages and monogamous relationships did not preclude HIV infection. Their constructions of marriage and the irony that ensued may come from the dominant discourses around intervening in HIV through the use of the ABCs. The "Be faithful" aspect of this intervention model, now widely used globally (although unsuccessfully), encourages couples to delay sex before marriage and to maintain monogamous relationships. One of the primary reasons this model and its admonition against promiscuity exists is because of funding guidelines from major financial sources like PEPFAR that are strongly grounded in ideological perspectives that promote abstinence and fidelity as central to their rules and regulations.

Although this point of view has been strongly criticized in discussions of the ABCs (see chapter 1) and even PEPFAR has eased some of its most conservative restrictions (see chapter 4), AB continues to be a focus of policy and scholarship around HIV. For example, recent trends in scholarship show a large number of studies blaming the spread of HIV on what is referred to as "concurrent sexual partnerships," meaning people who have multiple sex partners during the same general time period. This new term for an old way of thinking about HIV suggests that intervening in concurrent sexual partnerships is the way forward in HIV prevention. Because they are commonly conducted with black South Africans and black Americans, however, these kinds of studies wind up positioning black people as vectors of the virus and perpetuating racist myths about black promiscuity. They often conclude by calling for a greater focus on monogamy and faithfulness in interventions. In addition, they imply or even assert that some cultures (read black) are more accepting of concurrent sexual partnerships. Not only are these studies racist, but they also draw attention away from the fact that anti-concurrency campaigns have been largely unsuccessful and turn a blind eye to the fact that women in marriages and marriage-like relationships are actually more vulnerable to HIV.

Ultimately these discourses may have an impact on women like those we interviewed, who spoke frequently about the men in their lives. Castle (2004) states that HIV is a condition that is seen as having been imposed on people who have "transgressed social norms" (p. 13), whether it was inside or outside of the so-called safety net of marriage, and therefore deserve to be infected. People are encouraged, through discourses around faithfulness or through actual HIV intervention, to have a monogamous heterosexual partnership to prevent the spread of HIV. For women, this means there is a great emphasis on the necessity of having a man. Women may feel they have done something wrong in life to deserve HIV but that they can gain "redemption" and become a respectable person through men, marriage, and monogamy. Evidently, for the women we interviewed, marriage or a marriage-like relationship with a man acts as a barrier against the blame and stigma that HIV-positive women receive in society. As Lekas and her colleagues (2006) conclude from their research on stigma, one way these women cope with stigma is to emphasize something positive about themselves. In the interviews we conducted, the women choose to emphasize elements of their femininity. They draw on widespread discourses of "normalized femininity" in order to emphasize positive aspects of their living with HIV.

What about Love?

Another important issue related to HIV lies behind the intimate arrangements in which the women in our study live, and that is the question of emotional attachment. Marriage, and intimate relationships in general, increasingly includes the component of love. One of the important changes that developed in the social construction of marriage in the twentieth century is the importance of companionship and romantic love. Prior to that in the United States and Europe, marriage was primarily a financial arrangement. Among wealthy people it guaranteed that the heirs to a man's fortune were indeed his biological progeny. Among poor people, marriage was a way of bringing people and families together to consolidate tools, land, and other resources. Historians have documented changes in the ideas and experiences of marriage among middle-class white Americans that began at the turn of the twentieth century as people began to expect that their marriage would be a place to find love and that their spouse would be a life partner, a soul mate, and a romantic love (Mintz & Kellogg, 1988).

This idea of companionate marriage as an ideal appears to be part of many, if not most, societies all over the world today. The idea of love is now tightly linked to heterosexual partnerships as an essential component for many people, and "sexual intimacy is a key arena for the construction and demonstration of closeness" (Hirsch et al., 2009, p. 11). Because of these links, one would think that love would be a critical feature of scholarship on a sexually transmitted disease such as HIV. However, the emotional side of sex and HIV have been largely ignored, perhaps especially in reference to understanding HIV in Africa. "Whereas countless studies have analyzed how sexual behavior fuels the epidemic, few have explored how that behavior is embedded in emotional frameworks. Although the reduction of intimate relations to sex is problematic anywhere, this is especially the case for Africa because of the long history of Westerners deploying arguments of hypersexuality to dehumanize Africans and justify degrading policies" (Cole & Thomas, 2009, p. 4).

Mark Hunter (2010) writes that another related part of the reason for neglect of the emotional framework of HIV, particularly in Africa, is because of the invisibility in our thinking of the "materiality of everyday sex" (p. 4). He writes that love is intertwined in the exchange of material support and sex. Women and men engage in sexual relationships that also include gift giving. For example, historically, in the communities where he conducted his research in KwaZulu-Natal, a man provided *ilobolo,* or bridewealth, often in the form of cattle, as evidence of his emotional commitment to a woman. Today men may give women money, phone vouchers, rides, or food when they are involved in sexual relationships with women. Sometimes the exchanges are material transactions with little emotional connection and are a form of sex work or transactional sex. But often both the woman and man see themselves as intimately engaged sex partners who also give and take material support because they need it. "[S]ex is not simply exchanged instrumentally: the two lovers are 'boyfriend' and 'girlfriend,' not 'prostitute' and 'client'" (Hunter, 2010, p. 190). Hunter describes his findings in KwaZulu-Natal:

> The fact that they [relationships among young people in Mandeni] often involve gifts does not mean that they are not also loving: these relationships entangle love with gifts and sometimes violence. It is tempting to see highly material relationships as simply loveless; I did at first. But we must take more seriously the way people often understand their lives as simultaneously material and emotional despite, or perhaps precisely because of the existence of profound inequalities. (2010, p. 199)

Policy makers and scholars have tended to focus on these relationships as part of sex work and have not paid attention to the emotional connections and the ways couples understand love, sex, and gifts. Nevertheless, love is a critical component of the experience. Furthermore, love is socially constructed in ways that can bring emotional security and deeply positive feelings. Romantic love, however, has not proven to fulfill the promise of enhanced equity and intimacy that many women all over the world, including those in Africa, had hoped for (Smith, 2009). In fact, romantic love can create enormous risk and sacrifice if it is constructed as having sex without using condoms (Cole & Thomas, 2009). In addition, infidelity is also more difficult to confront, because marriages based on love are focused on the intimate couple as a unit rather than extended family or community, and therefore women are less likely to call on kin for support in the face of their husband's infidelity. Furthermore, if a woman's husband strays, she and those in her community may believe that he does not love her and that it is because she has failed as a lover and wife (Smith, 2009).

Relationships with men may be seen by the women we interviewed as advantageous because there may be a possible financial advantage to having a "man in the house." However, most of the women who participated in the present study are the breadwinners for their household, and their earnings often go toward taking care of children and men. Having a man around the house, therefore, must serve other purposes for women; one of these is to present their household and themselves as normal. As discussed earlier, stigma is a cruel and difficult aspect of being HIV positive, and the women we interviewed in Cape Town seek to overcome stigma by finding ways to present themselves as normal rather than as others. Work is one way they establish their normalcy and their value as members of the community. Having men partners, especially in marriage, is another significant way of claiming themselves a normal part of their families and the community.

Work and family are also aspects of femininity. As the women proclaim themselves normal through work and marriage, they also are establishing themselves as true women, fitting easily within the ideals of femininity in their community in South Africa. Having a man partner and marriage is associated with the social construction of femininity in many cultures, including the Cape Town Coloured community. Work is less often perceived as an essential aspect of femininity, but because of the legacy of apartheid and the continuing institutions of racism that require Coloured women to earn a living in the paid labor force, work is also an intrinsic feature of being a woman.

Finally, having a man partner provides women with what they have constructed as love, and with what the media and their friends and family tell them is love. They have a man who lives with them in an intimate partnership and who shows his feelings of closeness, companionship, and love in the most significant act: having sex with them. This strategy of embracing romantic love, however, has its downside as well (Cole & Thomas, 2009).

7 Care Work

THE WOMEN WE interviewed spoke frequently of work in general and about care work in particular. Many of the women in our study fear for their own day-to-day survival in terms of just finding enough food to eat and not suddenly dropping dead of HIV (several women expressed this as their greatest fear). Despite these real concerns about themselves, they also talked about taking care of their men partners and their children and worrying about the care work that remains undone. In the next chapter we will look at the care work women do for their partners and how that work often takes place in the context of violent relationships. This chapter focuses on the general issue of care work as it relates to people living with HIV and care work that the women in our study do for their children.

Care work is a central feature of nearly all women's lives, and it is a core component of the dominant versions of the social construction of femininity: emphasized femininities. In most societies, including South Africa, to be a woman is to be expected to do care work—in fact, to spend a lot of time providing care for others. The issue of care, not surprisingly, emerged as a significant discourse in our interviews. Care work was discussed in two related forms. First, the need for care is critical among people living with HIV; the women in our study reflected that need and the difficulties they face in finding, or, more often, not finding, adequate care. Second, the care work that women provide for their families is an important part of their lives and an essential aspect of how they construct themselves as women. For these women, constructing oneself as feminine and normal ideally includes living in an intimate relationship with a man and working for a living. Another feature of femininity that is central to the experience of the participants is taking care of others, especially the children and men in their lives. The issue of care work is one that emerged as a key factor in the discourse of women as they described their experience of HIV, the challenges they face, and their efforts to normalize themselves in spite of these challenges.

Care Work as Social Support

Many different terms are used to refer to various forms of care work. One of the terms frequently used in the HIV literature is "social support." However, this is a broad term, because there are many ways people living with HIV may receive social support (if they are indeed receiving any support at all). Although the term is difficult to define because it has been used in so many different ways by various scholars, Green (1993) offers a general definition of social support in the context of illness: "(i) the existence, quantity and type of interpersonal relationships (network structure or social interaction), (ii) the functional content of these relationships (emotional, psychological, tangible or informational support), and (iii) the perceived quality or adequacy of this support" (p. 90). All of these aspects of social support are part of the experience of people living with HIV.

People with chronic illnesses such as HIV sometimes receive different forms of social support from friends and family members, from support groups, and from social workers and health-care workers (Folkman, Chesney & Christopher-Richards, 1994; Friedland, Renwick & McColl, 1996; Green, 1993; Kelly & Mzizi, 2005; Schwarzer, Dunkel-Schetter & Kemeny, 1994). Social support from all of these sources has been found to contribute to quality of life. Good social support, regardless of the source, is said to have a buffering effect against the anxiety resulting from many of the challenges of living with HIV, including stigma (Servellen & Lombardi, 2005). In addition to aiding in emotional support and reducing fear and worry, this kind of comfort has critical implications for the health of those receiving the care. People who receive adequate social support from their health-care provider, for example, show better adherence to ARVs and other medication (Bakken et al., 2000; Catz, Heckman, Kochman & DiMarco, 2001; Chesney, 2003). Lower stress and better adherence to medication regimens result in improved physical health. People living with HIV who receive what they consider adequate support have higher CD4 counts and a longer survival rate (Ashton et al., 2005; Theorell et al., 1995).

As the prevalence of HIV increases, particularly for women, the need for care and social support increases, but care and support systems are oftentimes inadequate. In a study about the limitations of ARV programs in South Africa, Kelley and Mzizi (2005) found that simply making support groups available to people living with HIV is not enough. Sometimes circumstances make it difficult or impossible for people to attend such meetings. The barriers in accessing various forms of social care and support are varied and numerous. They include forms of HIV stigma and the inability to afford transport to support group meetings. These barriers and the resistance or inability of policy makers to strengthen and increase public care has meant that the vast responsibility of caring for people living with HIV has fallen to individual families and households.

Women Providing Care

The term "social support" is a general heading for the varied forms of support that are essential particularly for people who are living with HIV (or any chronic illness). The range of activities for which people living with the virus may require support include feeding, bathing, buying/finding food, cooking, cleaning, and many more. As we mentioned in chapter 2, the neighborhoods where our interviews took place are areas to which Coloured South Africans were removed during apartheid. They continue to live in these isolated areas that lack the most basic resources. People live in communities where indoor plumbing is scarce, gas or propane for stoves is unavailable, electricity is expensive, household appliances are beyond household budgets, and very few people own cars and cannot rely on public transport. In addition to daily household chores such as grocery shopping, cooking, cleaning, and washing clothes, people have other tasks. Many must collect water from a public tap because some dwellings do not have running water, and many must gather firewood from faraway fields and then haul the heavy fuel home on foot. Because large numbers of people do not have indoor plumbing, or their plumbing is in disrepair and too expensive to fix, even helping someone to the toilet means taking the person to wait in line at temporary outdoor toilets that the government has set up in long rows down main streets. If someone becomes gravely ill, there becomes even more work for care and support givers, including dressing wounds, providing assistance in walking, purchasing and administering medication, caring for children more often, supplementing household income, and the list goes on (Odgen, Esim & Grown, 2004). Although tasks like these are common and recognized as essential for the survival of individuals as well as economies, they are almost always unpaid (Makina, 2009).

In addition to care needed by adults and children who are living with HIV, there is also the issue of children whose parents are ill or who die as a result of HIV. UNAIDS (2010) estimates that there were 2.3 million children (under the age of 14) living with HIV in sub-Saharan Africa at the end of 2010. In addition, the organization estimates that there are about 14.8 million children (under the age of 18) in sub-Saharan Africa who have been orphaned because of AIDS. "AIDS orphans" is a term that has been disputed in the literature, since it has been documented that most "orphans" in sub-Saharan Africa live with a grandparent (Jones, 2005; UNICEF, 2006). Children whose parents die as a result of HIV often move into the households of grandparents, foster families, or others who are likely to be poor to begin with, stretching budgets even further and exacerbating economic problems. In addition, caring for children whose parents are too ill to do so or whose parents have died is most often done by the women in the households. Furthermore, caregivers receive little or no support from private or public institutions.

Earlier we mentioned that a number of terms are used to describe different types of support for people living with HIV that could all fall under the broad heading of social support, but this terminology leaves some important aspects of care work hidden. In an attempt to uncover those hidden aspects, Jessica Odgen and her colleagues (Ogden, Esim & Grown, 2004) coined the terms "linked" and "unlinked" care (p. 3). They assert that whether the care is emotional, practical, or medical is not the issue; the issue is whether or not the care work is provided by an individual who is linked to a funded organization or government unit and being paid and trained by that organization. Support groups, medical care, and other services provided by nongovernmental organizations (NGOs) are linked care work. The people who provide these services are trained and usually paid for their labor. Support groups and medical care alone, however, are not enough for those who fall ill or face other challenges because of HIV. There are more "everyday," omnipresent forms of support and care that need to be provided. These include the usual tasks of running a household plus the additional work that is necessary in communities and homes with few resources and very ill family members.

Despite the enormous amount of energy and skill involved in care work that is provided for "free" by family members for others, even for those who are ill and require special care, it is often thought of as a given or not "real work." In addition, care work is often thought of as work that comes "naturally" to some and not others. These ideas are related to the notion of gender essentialism, which is the belief that there is a true, in-born essence at the cores of men and women that makes them different from one another. One essentialist belief is that women are more nurturing and emotional than men for biological and physiological reasons, and that therefore women are more suited to activities that demand a nurturing personality or that they especially enjoy doing care work and are naturally skilled at doing it. Research by feminist scholars has overturned the validity of these essentialist beliefs about gender. Care work is indeed real, and although there is nothing inevitable or natural about the distribution of care work to women, it is women who actually do most of this work, especially unpaid care work, in nations all over the world.

In addition to being invisible and gendered, unlike linked/paid/formal work, this kind of work is never-ending—there is no "quitting time" (Elson, 2005). The work is relentless and unpaid, and it comes with a great cost to the provider (Harrington Meyer, Herd & Michel, 2000). Care and social support for people living with HIV, like all other care work, is fraught with these problems: it is relentless, undervalued, invisible, takes an enormous amount of physical and emotional energy, and it is assigned primarily to women.

Social support and caregiving for people living with HIV are costly for governments; they are especially burdensome in sub-Saharan Africa, where HIV prevalence is high and finances are low due to a long legacy of colonialism, apartheid, and global debt (Oxfam, 2007, February). One way that the South African government, like those of many other countries in the world, has been able to offset the cost of HIV care has been to cash in on this gendered nature of work. Policy makers have decided that because the formal sector is overburdened and informal, home-based care work appears to be free, governments must shift as much care work as possible to private families (Budlender, 2004). Since most of this care is done by women, the end result is that governments are shifting, or retaining, the responsibility for care work to unpaid women. Women are viewed as the natural-born caregivers within families, and families are viewed as being in the "private sphere," not to be tampered with by government policy and therefore not to be supported or paid by government programs. Although support and care work could potentially be provided by the state, instead the work has been easily outsourced to women in families and communities where people living with HIV require care (Makina, 2009).

This "solution" to the immense demands for care has led to a shift in the burden of care from governments that cannot or will not finance it to the women of each particular country. According to the Global Coalition on Women and AIDS, a UNAIDS initiative, nearly all (90 percent) of home care is provided by women (UNAIDS/UNFPA/UNIFEM, 2004). The women providing the care for people living with HIV are mothers, grandmothers, and girls (UNAIDS, 2004). These women may be family members, nurses, NGO workers, or community members and may or may not be living with the virus.

From the viewpoint of policy makers, this solution to the cost-of-care problem is ideal. In addition, there are possibly advantages to the person being cared for. Home-based care might be better for people who are ill, because they are surrounded by loved ones, are less likely to be exposed to infection as in a hospital setting, and do not have to deal with the stress and cost of traveling to and from the hospital or clinic (Avert, 2010c). In theory these benefits might be a conscious decision someone makes about their treatment, but in reality, especially for the marginalized, "being cared for at home is often an inevitability rather than a choice" (Avert, 2010c, p. 1). As Budlender (2004) explains, "policy makers often assume that there is a limitless supply—that they can have as much [unpaid HIV care work done by women] as they want" (p. 38), but there is a limit, there are major problems with this "solution," and there is certainly a cost for the women providing the care. Furthermore, if the care provided in homes is better for those receiving it, the work should be compensated.

In her study on gender and HIV, Urdang (2006) reviewed social support systems in southern Africa and found that women, rather than governments, were carrying the burden of care work for people living with HIV. She found that the care economy (including social support) for people living with HIV is almost all (90 percent) home-based and that the burden of responsibility for this care is disproportionately placed on women who may be living with HIV themselves and who are financially strapped. Urdang also points out that even some of the more formal or organized care and support programs are "organized around the assumption that nurturing is women's role and thus implicitly support patterns of female exploitation, even abuse" (p. 167). In the next chapter we will see how the link between nurturance and femininity results in women being tied to caring for men who are abusive and thus unable to leave violent relationships.

But abuse can take many forms and can be at the hands not only of violent partners but also of the social structure. Women who are forced to do care work because of social norms and the lack of any alternative care for themselves and their families are "abused" by a social context of poverty that makes their work inhumanely demanding. Women (who are often HIV positive themselves) struggle to provide care for family and community members living with HIV, and they must do this in an economic context that is difficult for everyone; this is especially so when family members are living with HIV. Their grocery bills are higher because they must buy special foods for HIV-positive family members, who must be particularly careful of nutrition. Their health-care costs are, of course, greater; transportation is more difficult and more expensive for people who are ill; and eventually they must pay for funerals and burials of those who die (UNAIDS, 2005). In addition, the household income may be reduced because those who are living with HIV are unable to work on a steady basis. Furthermore, those who are caring for those living with HIV may see smaller paychecks because of lost days at work. A study of South African households affected by HIV found that 40 percent of those surveyed had to take time off of work to care for someone living with HIV (Steinberg et al., 2002). In the South African context, taking time off of work is a great risk because of the intense competition for jobs. As the financial situation worsens in these situations, women who are living with HIV or are caring for people who are HIV positive must seek ways to earn money, including sex work, even if those ways are detrimental to their own health.

Dunkle and her colleagues (Dunkel et al., 2004), for example, studied people in Soweto, South Africa, who were engaged in transactional sex, a form of sex work in which the worker (usually a woman) does not identify as a sex worker but exchanges money or other resources such as food and transportation for sex. This form of sex work is a common method, often the only one, that a woman who is in dire need of money or other resources can use to acquire what she needs for herself and her family to survive (UNAIDS, 2005). Not only are women forced by limited options to engage in transactional sex because of the desperate situation they are in, but it is also nearly impossible for them to negotiate condom use in such transactions. For example, men who offer money, gifts, or other greatly needed resources may be willing to pay a higher price for sex without a condom—an offer that a woman in great need may not be able to turn down (Hallman, 2005).

The discussion thus far has focused on the gendered character of care work for women who are caring for people in their households who are living with HIV. Not only do women pay the cost of care for HIV, but younger girls do too. In a study in Zimbabwe, Mushunje (2006) found that when HIV-positive women who are doing care work fall too ill to continue with their household responsibilities, it is the girl child who usually takes over the tasks. When a girl's parents die as a result of HIV, not only does she suffer the tremendous grief of the traumatic loss, but she also must take on the burden of caring for the other children in her household. Girls are further oppressed in this situation because they are the first to drop out of school to become the sole breadwinner when they and their siblings are orphaned because of AIDS (Nyamukapa, Foster & Gregson, 2003). Not only are the girls prevented from continuing their education, because they are even less likely to find legitimate paid work than are adults in these circumstances, but they are often forced to engage in transactional sex as the only income-generating opportunity available. Like the older women who have little chance of exercising any control over condom use, these girls are even more vulnerable to becoming infected by HIV. Because of their youth and their lack of choices, they are even less able to negotiate condom use and therefore more likely to be exposed to HIV. In addition, their younger, smaller bodies are more physiologically vulnerable to damage during intercourse and therefore more likely to become infected with STIs, including HIV.

Doing Care Work for Children

As we will see in the next chapter, the women we interviewed described the care work they did for men as eliciting very little care in return. Unlike the care work done for the men in their lives, the investment of time and energy in care work the women do for their children may have a material return. Sometimes women are able to benefit from care work done for children because their children in turn learn to care for their mothers. The caring the women do for children is reciprocal. Other scholars have found, for example, that children whose mothers are HIV positive have a lot to do with the decisions women make about their lives, and that children play a positive role in encouraging and helping their mothers adhere to using ARVs (Wood, Tobias & McCree, 2004). In our study we found that some children take an active, positive role in this regard. In addition, in some families women are particularly determined to equip their children with skills for care work, because they know they need the help.

The challenge of providing what they believe to be adequate care for their children causes the women much anxiety. The women's ability to care for their children in ways that meet conventional expectations about femininity, especially mothering, or even to provide for their children's basic needs is often nearly impossible. Their failure to meet these impossible goals is a contributing factor to stress levels and an ultimate decline in overall health. Nevertheless, for many women, the benefits—or necessities—outweigh the risks to health, and the women continue to struggle to try to provide care for their children. The care work the women do keeps their children alive. Furthermore, the women believe that doing care work, especially if it is successful, allows them to continue to think of themselves as "decent" women and loving wives and mothers. Care work thus operates to neutralize stigma and fend off the marginalization women are confronted with because they are living with HIV along with various other oppressive forces in their lives. Care work is also a measure of a woman's normalcy and health. If an HIV-positive woman is still attending to the needs of others, she can think of herself as not yet entirely overwhelmed by HIV and not yet completely defined by her HIV status.

Stories of Caring for Children

Priscilla is a woman with considerable worries about taking care of her children when she "finally gets sick." Priscilla began talking about caring for her children in response to our first interview question about when she first found out she was living with HIV.

> I've got four kids, the eldest one is 15, and 10 and 6 years and 2 years old—
> I don't know what's gonna happen to them, you know? There's a lot of things
> on my mind. Every time I just think, "Oh, God! What's gonna happen to them
> when I'm dying?" Because this illness is . . . I don't know, Anna, but my wor-
> ries here is I'm going to get sick—I know I'm going to get sick, and I ask God
> to fight and to keep me strong, because I don't know what's gonna happen to
> them—especially to my baby.

Later in the interview Priscilla emphasized again her stress about not being able to provide properly for her children, especially her oldest daughter.

> I would like to earn something because I got a 15-year-old daughter, you
> know, Anna, she wants pants for Christmas. I don't have that kind of money.
> It's R 750 [US$100]. I don't have that money. Because her friends are wearing
> names [brands], you know. And she don't understand.

Priscilla feels that because of her HIV status, which has led to her inability to find a decent job, she is unable to provide for her children properly. She repeatedly cited this as one of her greatest sources of anxiety.

Elaine also talked about taking care of her children. She explained one of the reasons she decided to go on ARVs despite hearing horror stories about them: her children will have a difficult time surviving if she is not there to care for them. Although her work caring for them is invisible, she knows that she must continue to do it as long as possible. And she believes that the ARVs will allow her to live a little longer. Here she relays what she said to her sister, who is a nurse and was warning her against taking ARVs: "I've got children that I must look after. Nobody's looking after my children. Who's gonna look after my children?"

Not only does Elaine worry about her children not being cared for at all if she dies, but she also talked about how she is often unable to provide the care they need. She described her struggles to buy or find food for her children.

> Even at home also—if there's no money, there's food. I don't worry. As long as I've got food in the house, I don't worry. Why must I worry? The children ask me, "Mommy, what are we gonna eat tonight?" I say, "We just eat that what is there. If you must eat potatoes, you just eat potatoes."

Although Elaine says, "Why must I worry?" clearly she is worried about providing food, because she tells her children they must eat what is available, if anything is available at all.

Elaine also spoke about care work as it involves her children caring for her in return. Here she told us about when she disclosed her positive status to her children. When her youngest daughter began to cry, Elaine explained how it was no time to cry, but to begin learning how to do care work.

> Mommy's not gonna die. If Mommy gets sick, Mommy must go to the hospital, to the clinic. This is Mommy's tablets that Mommy must use. Mommy mustn't forget to drink these tablets. *If* [she emphasizes] Mommy forget, you must remember Mommy every time, "Did Mommy drink tablets, or did Mommy not?" Then will Mommy drink and Mommy will tell you okay. Or Mommy forgot something and then you must come and remind me.

In the above excerpt, Elaine reviews the steps to caregiving with her daughter, teaching her a caregiver's duties. Her experience was not unique. A number of women we interviewed spoke about teaching their daughters to do care work, although their efforts have not always been successful.

Stress and Tensions for Mothers and Children

The mothers in our study spoke about frustrations they have with their daughters and how HIV has created or exacerbated problems in their relationships with their children, their daughters in particular. The women's ways of speaking about their children, especially their daughters, with regard to caring for them and the problems they face in doing so were revealing, but they only tell half of the story. Interviews were not conducted with the daughters themselves, so we have only the perceptions of these mother-daughter encounters from the mothers' point of view.

Schrimshaw and Siegel's (2002) study on what happens when mothers who are HIV positive disclose their status to their children illustrates the differing reactions children have. Some of the children in their study reacted by becoming closer to their mothers; others reacted negatively, blaming their mothers and exhibiting behavioral problems. Our interviews, too, revealed contradictions and mixtures of women's reliance on their children for emotional and physical support alongside failures in getting their children to help them or even to treat them humanely. Several women spoke at length about their attempts at teaching their daughters to do care work and how their attempts have been riddled with obstacles.

Sonia struggles to take care of her children. Her oldest daughter resents her for this and for contracting HIV, but here she speaks about the care work that her second-oldest daughter is learning to do.

> My eldest daughter, we have so much problems I can't ask her to be my treatment buddy [treatment buddies are chosen by those who are taking ARVs to ensure their adherence to treatment by directly observing them swallowing medication in the correct dosage at the right time]. . . . Would you believe me, Anna, if I tell you that Delia [her second-oldest daughter] is reminding me when we at home, every day, "Did you drink your tablets? Did you drink your tablets? . . ." I mean. She's 13 years old and she's reminding me, and, and that is the thing that my eldest daughter should be training herself to do already.

Above, Sonia relates how her second-oldest daughter knows her "duties" as a caregiver in making sure her mother has taken her tablets. Sonia feels frustrated not only with the fact that her eldest daughter is not caring for her, but also that she cannot provide and care for her daughters in the ways she would like to. She reiterated this point when she answered the question of what her greatest fear or worry is since being diagnosed.

> My biggest fear is that I should die without making proper provision for my children. Because I'm now in a very, very cheap burial society that's the PEP insurance at the PEP stores [PEP stores are a local department store chain that has cashed in on the HIV pandemic by selling relatively cheap burial insurance in South Africa]. I don't have additional insurance to fall back on. Umm, my children isn't in a proper house; umm, their education I'm also worried about, because anything can happen; umm, who is gonna be my little one's guardians if I should die before they the age of consent; umm, who's gonna be my treatment buddy when I must go on ARVs. Umm, all that type of fears I know . . . I also have my fears. That's—that's my fears.

Sonia has listed her duties as a caregiver. She asserts that arrangements for her children's housing, education, and future guardians need to be made. She even worries about her own burial. But for all of these responsibilities she has very little support. She lists these duties in the form of an inventory of her "fears," because they are seemingly impossible to allay given her circumstances.

Denise also expressed severe anxiety over her inability to care for her children as she sees necessary. Denise is unable to find steady work and has been fired from jobs because she falls ill (literally, because she has frequent fainting spells) and has to leave work and take days off to visit doctors. Here she explains how she is unable to care for her daughter in some very basic ways.

> Everything is difficult . . . everything is difficult because I can't do . . . sometimes we sleep without food . . . because that's why because she is not in school . . . sometimes the children are at home . . . and then this year I didn't

pay school fees for her . . . I didn't do anything. . . . Lot of things, lot of things . . . what am I going to eat today, how my child is gonna go to school, plus I don't have money for transport. You see? How am I going to wash my washing [laundry], just like that?

Denise's language usage above, such as the repetition of "everything is difficult" and "lot of things," illustrates her feelings of being overwhelmed with her difficulties and the despair of her situation. She explains that she is not even able to provide her daughter with basic needs like schooling because of the expense. In South Africa free K–12 state schools do exist but are not accessible to all children because of the high cost of public transport. South Africans pay R 8,000–R 20,000 (US$1,100–2,700) per year for state-aided K–12 schools, or between R 30,000–R 70,000 (US$4,000–9,300) per year for private K–12 schools (Southafrica.info, 2012). These fees are far beyond Denise's reach, so her daughter cannot attend school, and Denise agonizes about her inability to provide sufficient care for her child.

Denise has also attempted to teach her oldest daughter to help in the care work she needs, but to no avail. Her 16-year-old daughter is her greatest worry, because she refuses to do housework and it is possible that she is having unprotected sex with her boyfriend.

DENISE: And it's only me and my daughter.

ANNA: Does your daughter help you?

DENISE: She like to be on the street . . . She don't even like to cook—she's— she's 16! She's turning 17 this year October . . . Worried about what my daughter's doing. Bringing the boyfriend in the house. Sleeping with the boyfriend in the house. You understand that?

ANNA: Has anyone ever helped you with any of those problems?

DENISE: No. No people just talk behind me. Can't tell me straight. "She let that boyfriend in the house . . ." I don't—I don't like it . . . just because I don't like to talk because she's gonna say I'm giving her a difficult life. You understand? She don't understand this . . . she—she [crying] you know, stressing me.

Denise has tried to teach her daughter to perform care work, but her daughter has resisted. In addition, her description of her daughter "be[ing] on the street" is especially significant, since Denise is telling us that she feels she has not provided sufficient care for her daughter because she unable to make her abide by community expectations about young women.

In extensive research with people in Manenberg, which is an area of forced removal near the community where our study took place, Elaine Salo (2002) explains how women who are frequently seen outside the home are seen as improper or "loose." Salo describes the importance of mothers policing their daughters' sexuality with the hopes that "the daughters internalize these policing strategies, so that they [regulate] their own sexuality" (p. 410–411). She says that without this sort of policing, a household's "moral reputation" and "sexual reputation" may suffer, and it may be the case that "one's moral reputation spell[s] the difference between continued hardship and relief" (p. 409).

Denise believes it may be impossible to convince her daughter to help her, because her daughter resents her and feels that Denise has "given her a difficult life." Denise is scared for her daughter's well-being as well as her own, but she says she has come to the end of her rope. She cries when she speaks about the problems she has with her daughter, but she also speaks in a very dejected way and has mentioned leaving her children and relinquishing the job of caregiver to her best friend or grandmother.

Some women describe problems they have had in providing their daughters with basic necessities and their daughters' negative reactions to this. In the discussions with the women we interviewed and in the casual conversations we had with several of their daughters, we found that some of the daughters resent their mothers for becoming HIV positive (field notes, January 2007). This blaming and resentment is a reaction seen in other studies of South African women living with HIV as well. Schrimshaw and Siegel (2002) note that some children see their mothers as responsible for the "mess" that they are all now in. The daughters of the women in our study are especially critical of their mothers' continued caring for or being involved with men who are detrimental to their lives (and who may have infected their mothers). As much as the mothers want their daughters to conform to the caregiving role, the daughters continue to resist. Sometimes this is beneficial to the daughters because it means they are not shouldering as great a burden. But sometimes it works to their disadvantage when it exacerbates the household's problems or threatens their relationships with their mothers.

Femininity and Care Work in Cape Town

Salo's (2005) research in Manenberg, a neighborhood in Cape Town similar to the one where our interviews were conducted, illustrates the gender norms in a Coloured community in South Africa where older women teach their daughters acceptable gendered behavior. These expectations include behaving in modest ways in terms of dress; venturing outside the house only if accompanied by an older woman or if some appropriate task is to be done; and taking responsibility for domestic chores (which includes care work). Salo goes on to explain that these gender expectations for women are starting to erode as young women search for new identities (for better or worse) in postapartheid South Africa. These findings may be related to some of the problems the women we interviewed related concerning their daughters. Not only do daughters and mothers renegotiate their relationships with each other as a result of the mother's HIV, but they also undertake these renegotiations in a context in which gender is changing and their beliefs and values contrast and conflict with those of the other generation.

Taking care of daughters in particular is a struggle in that these young women are resistant and wary of repeating the patterns of their mothers, and they place blame on and stigmatize their mothers and the virus the mothers are living with. There is an element of hope, however, because although the daughters may not always be doing what is best for themselves and their mothers, at least they are resisting. It is important to note that although the possible resistance of hegemonic gendered behaviors on the part of daughters is a positive step, it is not a justification for the blame and stigma that they may place on their mothers. Nevertheless, there are indeed daughters who are resisting or rebelling against their mothers and, in doing so, are rejecting some of the gender hierarchies that have failed their mothers.

The dilemma women face in providing care and social support is complicated by the economic context in which they live, a context that has emerged from an apartheid past and from the continued inequities and economic challenges that persist. It is also shaped by the dependence of governments on the invisible and unpaid care work that keeps individuals and families alive (albeit barely in many cases). And it is affected by the expectation that it is women who must provide the care work even if they are the ones in the greatest need of care. The women we interviewed explained how they must care for men and children while many times enduring acts of abuse at the hands of the men for whom they are caring. The women are compelled to perform and emphasize their gendered duties of "self-sacrificer" and "caregiver," often to the detriment of their own health and well-being, in order to perform necessary care work and to provide evidence that they are "proper" women despite the fact that they are living with HIV. The ways women speak about care work done for both their man partners and their children indicate that the hegemonic constructions of gender that women rely on for acceptance and survival are not working. Unfortunately, this normalizing tool is a strategy by which an overarching system of male dominance and gender injustice keeps women in their place and legitimizes their oppression and abuse. Their daughters in some cases are seeking to challenge these constructions of gender. Ironically, however, in doing so these young women may be helping to bring down the system of gender injustice while simultaneously causing their mothers a great deal of grief just when they are most in need of support.

8 Care Work and Violent Men

CHAPTER 7 DESCRIBED the problems with care work that women do, especially for their children, but problems also exist in the care work they do for the men in their lives. Ironically, the discussion of care work for men in our interviews with the women was mostly talk about men within a context of abuse. The women are caring for men partners, despite their own HIV-related problems and, even more surprisingly, despite the abuse inflicted upon them by the men for whom they are caring. Women drew on discourses of femininity in describing how men need their care, even in abusive situations. Some of the women acknowledged that being a "proper wife," which includes caring for men's sexual needs, has taken a toll on their physical health, yet they continue not only to live with their male partners but also to take care of them. The following excerpts illustrate the women's struggles to take care of men, many times in the midst of an abusive relationship.

HIV Infection and Partner Violence

Shareen's trouble started when she got married, two years before we interviewed her. A short time into the marriage she found out about her husband's positive HIV status when she visited him in the hospital. She had taken the liberty of reading his medical chart at the foot of his bed, which listed him as being HIV positive. Once she learned that he had tested positive, she believed it was necessary to have herself tested for the virus. She explained to us how painful it was to get tested secretly and alone while he was in the hospital.

> I go on the 14th of December, and the doctor took my finger and he didn't say—the sister didn't tell me I'm HIV the same time. She told me I must go to the other room with my file, and I see on her face there is something not right. And she asked me, "Shareen, if I told you you are HIV, how would you feel?" I didn't talk . . . I told the sister, "But you must tell me now the truth if I'm HIV or not." And she say to me, "Shareen, you are HIV positive." [pause] And I sit there and I hold my head, and I take my hair and I do like this [pulling] and I put my head against the wall. And I start crying, crying, crying.

Shareen lives with an abusive husband. She described what happened after she found out that she, too, was HIV positive. In the days after being told her status by the nurse, she decided it was important to avoid becoming pregnant, because she did not want to risk transmitting HIV to her baby. Before she could get an appointment for birth control at the clinic, however, Shareen learned that she already was pregnant. She then tried to get an abortion but was refused at the clinic on the grounds that her husband was not present for the procedure.

South Africa's Choice on Termination of Pregnancy Act of 1996 states that "no consent other than that of the pregnant woman shall be required for the termination of a pregnancy" (p. 3). According to this law, Shareen had the right to terminate her pregnancy without permission from her husband (or anyone else), but the health-care providers at the clinic chose not to abide by the law. If Shareen had been aware of her legal rights, she might have been able to challenge the clinic in time to proceed with the abortion. Even then, however, it would have taken much time and resources to question their rule. In addition, because she has a low income and lives in a somewhat isolated community, finding another health-care provider would be difficult. And, in any event, she had no reason not to believe the personnel at the first clinic when they told her that her husband must be present.

Despite the apparent injustice of being prevented from terminating her pregnancy, Shareen explained that she now believes the unexpected pregnancy has benefited her.

> My husband was very happy. [pause] Because I had . . . for, for, for a year and two months my . . . my life wasn't right. Every two days my husband hit me. And now the baby's here and he's happy, and he don't hit me anymore.

When Shareen finally confronted her husband, he admitted to having known his status for a long time. His family also knew about his status, and she questioned them as well on a trip to visit them in another province.

> I ask his mother why she didn't tell me that her son was HIV positive. She told me if she gonna tell me, I'm gonna drop [leave] her son. I say, "No, I don't wanna drop. I also now have the same virus he have." And now my mother-in-law told me if I don't want her son anymore about this, she don't want—I must go and leave—I must leave. I say, "No, I love him. I'm staying here by him. Fight with this together." She say, "Okay, if you're like this, you can stay."

Here it is important to explain not only the words Shareen says but also the manner in which she spoke about these upsetting events. She talked quietly and without expression as if she has become numb. In spite of the distressing incidents of receiving a positive HIV test, being infected by someone who knew his status and claimed to love her but did not inform her or take precautions to protect her from infection, being kept ignorant by other family members who knew of his status, being illegally refused an abortion, and being physically abused, Shareen has decided to stay with her husband, who is frequently ill, and "fight this together." Her description of the behavior of her partner's family, who did not tell her he was living with HIV, shows how social bonds beyond the immediate partnership can tie women to violent men. Religious beliefs are also pertinent to her decision. Shareen considers herself a religious person and claims this has shaped her think-

ing and behavior with regard to her husband. Shareen is undoubtedly also staying with her physically abusive husband because there is nowhere else for her to
live. But she justifies her decision by emphasizing her belief in the notion of religious forgiveness for the abuse, which may be an additional force that is drawing
her even closer to her husband (Boonzaier & de la Rey, 2004).

Because Shareen's husband is quite ill, she may also be telling us that care work
for dependent men is a behavior expected of women and therefore one that she
expects of herself. From a feminist point of view, these expectations or forced behaviors are essential aspects not only of the maintenance and support of the dominance of individual men over their women partners but also of an ongoing system
of masculine hegemony and the subordination of women, and subsequently the
justification of woman abuse (Dobash & Dobash, 1979). Because of the way oppressive gender expectations have been constructed for women living in a masculine-
dominated society, caregiving is a type of work women are compelled to do, for
the survival of others as well as for acceptance in society. In fact, many women
across the globe define themselves, at least in part, by their ability to satisfy gender expectations for women by providing care and putting the needs of others before their own (Gunsaullus, 2006).

Priscilla was also infected by a partner who was aware of his positive status be-
forehand but continued to have unprotected sex with her without telling her that
he was HIV positive. She told us about her partner's blasé, almost cheerful, attitude toward her positive HIV test.

> So he asked me, what did the doctors say, you know, with a smile on his
> face . . . And I was so scared to tell him, because I thought he's gonna leave
> me—maybe it's me with the virus, whatever . . . But my main problem was,
> "You gave it to me! You gave it to me!" And, umm, I talked to him, "I'm HIV
> and . . ." You know I didn't talk to him like I'm talking to you now. I was
> screaming and yelling and crying in between . . . and he said, "Oh, well, accept
> it Priscilla, because there's nothing that anyone can do . . . but I'm gonna show
> you how much I love you," and he make love to me without a condom.

Priscilla spoke of this incident repeatedly (field notes, August 2006), and in
these conversations she reiterated the fact that she did not want to have sex without a condom at that time. Significantly, she refers to the event as "making love
to me," which suggests that she is constructing the event in a manner that makes
her the submissive and passive party in the incident. These constructions of "male
sexuality as active" and "female sexuality as passive" by women who are in abusive relationships were also evident in the Boonzaier and de la Rey (2004, p. 458)
study. Additionally, her labeling the incident as "making love" (which sounds like
it is describing consensual sex) further reflects the findings in the Boonzaier and
de la Rey study in that women may be reluctant to label violent incidents like this
as rape. This may be because women in marriages or other types of marriage-

like relationships give in to their partners or feel they are obligated to be sexually available to them at all times.

Although Priscilla defended her decision to stay with her husband, she continued to speak of the physical and psychological abuse she has endured with her current partner. She also described her distress over her partner's refusal to discuss the fact that he knowingly infected her, how he became infected with HIV in the first place, and her attempts to make sense of his behavior.

> Because I just wanna know who gave it to me, that's all. You know I read last night a *Drum* [a magazine that emerged as part of the antiapartheid movement and has remained popular especially among people of color in South Africa]— it's not time to blame each other about this virus . . . if you find out you have this virus, just accept it. Don't blame him. Don't blame her. That is what I read in the *Drum*. But I don't know, Anna . . . I just . . . I think I just need some answers . . . You know, Anna, if you don't even tell me about the virus, then don't talk to me. He don't talk to me . . . He just lay in the bed, give his back to me . . . Don't talk to me. And I think that is also the problem, because he don't talk to me, Anna.

Priscilla's partner's abuse of her takes many forms, including rape, psychological cruelty, and infidelity. It also takes the form of physical assault and violence to the point of attempted murder. In our discussion she described an incident when her partner became intoxicated and tried to kill her so that he could be with another woman.

ANNA: Has he ever been violent?

PRISCILLA: Yes . . .

ANNA: What did he do?

PRISCILLA: He was drinking and he locked the door and he wanna . . . what is that? . . . how do you call that? . . . I don't know what do you call that in English, that you cut a hole? . . . Not a hammer . . .

ANNA: A saw?

PRISCILLA: Yes, a saw. He locked the door and then he tried to saw me [laughing]. Honestly, Anna.

ANNA: Did he cut you?

PRISCILLA: No.

ANNA: But he tried to saw you?

PRISCILLA: Yes, because Nazeem [the support group facilitator] was there to come and fetch me. Not last year . . . the year before.

ANNA: Why did he . . . because he was drunk or . . . ?

PRISCILLA: He was drunk and I think he got [was seeing] someone else, but I was in the way. So I told Nazeem he must come and fetch me. And he came and fetched me, and he took me to my sister. And he never drank again. That was the last. It isn't so, you know . . . so cute. There's also problems.

Priscilla has expressed great anxiety about all of the forms of emotional and physical abuse she experiences from her partner. But she is especially concerned about her need to know how she became infected with HIV and how her husband's infidelity resulted in her own infection.

The idea that infidelity is a form of woman abuse is an idea that has only recently begun to be explored by scholars. Boonzaier (2005) noted the emergence of infidelity as a form of control and abuse in her interviews with women in South Africa, and women in our own study frequently mentioned infidelity on the part of their partners as a major source of anxiety and as a possible reason for their positive HIV status. For the women we spoke with, infidelity is in itself an abusive act, but it also becomes even more harmful because it results in transmission of HIV from unfaithful men to the women. This reasoning is supported by the findings of Dunkle and her colleagues (2004) in research they conducted in Soweto that women who report abuse in their most recent relationships with men are more likely to be living with HIV. There are strong links among woman abuse, infidelity, and infection of women in intimate relationships with men who are abusive. Priscilla's story illustrates the dynamics of these links. It also illustrates the difficulty women have in extricating themselves from those relationships.

Abusive Partners Get Second Chances

In another segment of the interview, Priscilla described how both her partner and her daughter work to prevent her from leaving. Priscilla has tried to end the relationship each time her partner leaves her for a few days to be with other women. Here she explains their on-again, off-again relationship and some of the social forces that prevent her from leaving.

Every time he told me he's got someone better than me—then I put him out. Then he comes back. Every time it goes like this. On and off, on and off. So I told him, "No, man. It can't go on like this. I'm getting older, my kids are getting bigger. I think you must go." And I put him out, and I took his stuff and I threw it out. So he went. He go and two months ago, he came back to me. He crawled and cried and pleaded, "Please, Priscilla, take me back. Please? I'm asking you nicely." I mean, Anna, I was feeling so ashamed, you know? I asked my daughter, "Can Mommy give Darryl another chance?" So she said, "God gives you another chance, so why . . . but this is his last chance. Mommy just tell him."

Although these experiences appear to warrant leaving the relationship, the women we interviewed are in a predicament that is complicated by their marginalization. Like many abused women, their attempts to break away from abusive partners may be impossible because of threats of physical harm as well as other forms of manipulation. Their partnerships are also part of a web of social relations, and their individual decision to leave can be thwarted by the other ties that bind them. Furthermore, they may not be able to sacrifice the social "privileges" associated with having a man, especially when these women are already marginalized because they are living with HIV. For these reasons, the women are forced to embrace hegemonic, oppressive constructions of gender in hopes of legitimizing the abusive relationships.

Like Shareen, Priscilla is also willing to give her partner more chances. When Priscilla spoke about him, she expressed hatred, but it was mixed with pity and empathy, as both she and her partner are experiencing many of the same physical and emotional problems related to the HI virus. The way in which the women we interviewed talked about their HIV-positive status projects a kind of romanticized version of living with the virus and staying with the partner who is abusive and from whom she became infected. But it also reflects the observation made by third-wave feminist scholars that black women may not want to leave poor black men, even when their relationships are not satisfying, because the women see themselves as under the same threats as the men and therefore comrades in arms. The women in our study share this point of view and are even more strongly attached to the men in their lives, because they share the stigma as well as physical challenges of living with HIV.

Elvyra has also been abused by her husband. She reunited with her ex-husband thirty years after divorcing him. Her husband has known about her status all along, but he refuses to get tested or use condoms. Here she explains the problems he has with condoms.

> So we got married and we living together now. And so I said to him, "Anyway, I don't want you also to get sick, because then we both is gonna get sick. We can't look after each other. Either you must use a condom . . ." So he said, no, he's not gonna use a condom . . . he's not gonna use a condom . . . Anyway sometimes . . . then I ask him, "Are you sure you don't want to use a condom because maybe you want to . . . you must go for a test?" So he said, no, why must he go for a test, because he loves me and he wants to be with me, and why must he . . . why must he use a condom.

In the above quote, Elvyra draws on the dominant discourses of "getting tested" and "using condoms" that she has learned in her training as a peer counselor for HIV-positive people. Despite her training, however, she has been unable to convince her husband to take action for the sake of their own health.

A new report by the One in Nine Campaign (2012) shows that men are now more and more reluctant to test for HIV and are using their woman partners as a "test" for their own HIV status. Once a woman's status is confirmed (i.e., positive), men assume that they are positive too and share the medication women may have received. Not only does this create huge problems in terms of treatment and drug resistance, but it also means that women are sacrificing their health in order to take care of men partners. Elvyra's husband's refusal to be tested or use condoms endangers Elvyra's health further, and he also uses his refusal to use condoms as emotional leverage in the frequent arguments they have.

> Yes, sometimes we say words to each other, but there are sometimes he say he offered his life for me. That I can't understand, because now the other day I told him, "You were told. It's not to say that I didn't tell you. At first I told you about my status. It's your choice, so why did you stay? So don't come and throw it in my face now, because it's not gonna work." . . . Every time . . . maybe if we get an argument. Every time then he will just say, "I offered my life for you."

Elvyra's husband is inflicting various forms of abuse on her in his nonuse of condoms and in his refusal to get tested for HIV. His behavior allows him to be able to keep her in the dark, within his control, and indebted to him. Even worse, when he says that he has "offered his life," he turns the relationship upside down by constructing himself as the victim and Elvyra as the ungrateful exploitative partner. Violent men constructing themselves as victims is a common strategy men use to displace blame from themselves to their partner (Boonzaier & de la Rey, 2004). Elvyra's partner elaborates on his reversal of their relationship by maintaining that not only is he a victim of her ingratitude but that she has infected him with HIV and he is the victim of her body's disease. He does not acknowledge that he has forced her to expose him to HIV by refusing to use condoms with her. In this way he presents himself as a martyr and Elvyra as "diseased," and therefore he should take the upper hand in any disagreements, as he is morally superior.

Elvyra to some extent has bought into his reasoning and responds to her husband's blame by feeling indebted to him for wanting to be with her in spite of her illness. She also related, however, that these interpersonal tensions between them are not the only factor in her decision to stay with him. Taking him back despite the opinions of the rest of her family also has practical relevance, as she believes that he provides material support. This belief is not entirely based on fact; she contradicted this idea later in her interview when she said he is not working, provides no material support, and is a drug addict using her money to buy illegal drugs for himself. Elvyra said she initially left her husband because he was abusive. Now she talks about her family's reaction to their recent reunion.

> They knew him at that time that he was . . . he was very weird at that time. He was abusing me at that time . . . Maybe I think they disappointed because I take my ex-husband back that I got now. They are very disappointed, I think that. Because at the end of the day, who will support me? Will they support me? I mean he's working in the house. He's helping me. He put food on the table—are *they* gonna do it? But they never come to me and ask, "Elvyra, how are you feeling? I hear you sick . . ." or so.

In spite of what Elvyra describes as a deep need for her sisters to return their affections to her, she has chosen her husband over her family. She claims this is because of the care and financial support he offers, but later in the interview she described another reason for her choice.

> Yeah, because at this moment I also got stress. And, umm . . . because my husband is smoking drugs [methamphetamine]. And you know if he brings money home every time he asks me, "Give me money," also. But I just pray that I don't want to upset myself anymore or work myself up, because then I'm gonna be down . . . I'm attending a campaign now. At the moment it's on Sunday nights. So the pastor's helping me pray . . . that he [Elvyra's husband] must leave the drugs. We are on that now. On his case. Because that's all stress I've got now. At the moment . . . he want money now or they must smoke now. And that I can't take. And then I just say, "Here's a 20 Rand [about US$3]. Just go smoke, but leave me out. Because I want to rest. I want to read my Bible or take a class or something."

What Elvyra says here contradicts her earlier reasoning when she claimed she was staying with her husband because of the support he provides. Here she shows that the exact opposite is true. When we look at all of the explanations she gives for why she stays with her husband, it seems that the most important reason is because he is in need and she is able to offer him the care and support that he needs.

Elvyra has seemingly chosen to look after her husband—her former (and current) abuser—who now has an expensive addiction. In the next section of the interview, it was revealed that her choice is at the cost not only of increased anxiety and decreased social support from her family but also of her own fragile physical health.

> We *mos* [Afrikaans for "really"] seldom get shingles, right? Seldom that you get shingles. In last year, late in last year I had this stress from this husband of mine. So my whole body was full of shingles. I didn't sleep for three months. So I went to the day hospital [clinic]. So the doctor just lift up my top. So he said, "My good grief! Elvyra, how did you sleep, because this is a painful thing!" So they bandaged me from here till here [indicating her waist to under her breasts].

Elvyra has also taken on the responsibility of caring for her husband and attending prayer groups for the sake of her husband, who was and still is abusive to her. Taking care of her husband—because husbands are constructed as partners with whom women must stay, endure abusive treatment from, and care for—takes precedence over other issues in Elvyra's life. Women in previous studies (Urdang, 2006) as well in our own feel that in order to maintain their identity as good women and good wives they must take care of men partners and husbands, even if the man is abusive and even if the woman can point to specific ways that her health is suffering because of the care work she is doing.

Sonia is married but separated from her husband. She avoided speaking about why she is separated from her husband, mentioning only that they split during her pregnancy with their child, who is now eight years old and living with the virus as well. She hinted about his obsessiveness and jealousy and talked about having taken him back several times against her better judgment.

> Like with my boyfriends, I have a rule. I didn't tell them. I give them three chances and once okay, and twice okay, I forgive. Third time? Gone. My husband got seven because he's my husband. I gave him seven chances. He blew all seven chances.

Despite the nature of the problems they may have had, she explains her choice to continue to offer support to her husband. Sonia's use of the term "husband" is specific and significant. She has constructed her husband as quite different from a partner or boyfriend in that she may be required to, or it is legitimate to, give him "more chances" and endure so much more.

Below, Sonia describes an activity in one of the support groups she attends. The exercise was one in which each member had to stand beneath a photo that represents their feelings. This was the day she decided that she could not abandon her husband completely.

> And, and it was very heart-sore. And I think that's why I'm still so close to my husband, because he's also positive. I'm not sure if I gave it to him or if he had it before—that I will never know, but he was sick when I met him. And, umm, in any case . . . the thing is they were standing around and he went to go stand by the picture . . . the mother, the father, and the child separate. And I knew there and then that I couldn't leave him like that—irrespective how I feel about him, he's my brother. In spirit he's my brother and I can't desert him. I can divorce him, I can do whatever, but I can't desert him. So that's why I won't— I don't think I will ever be able to break that bond with my husband. He wants more. He wants me to be back with him and that, but I . . . I'm not up for that.

Although Sonia expressed an interest in being interviewed, she left out certain parts of her life in the interview, and it was not clear whether or not her decision to not "desert" her husband has been at a cost to her emotionally or physically. Nevertheless, she has taken back into her care a man who "blew it" seven times, and she describes it as an act of sympathy and love. Sonia speaks of the sympathy she feels toward her HIV-positive partner as well as seeing a need to care for him, saying she "can't desert him." Perhaps her husband would have neither psychological nor material support without her. As in the Boonzaier and de la Rey (2004) study, the way women speak about their sympathy and their need to do care work for their partners, shows that the line between "wife" and "mother" has become blurred. It also shows that the construct of mother implies unconditional love and caregiving for those who are her "children."

Elaine also spoke about caring for a person who was previously abusive to her. She had an ex-boyfriend who took advantage of her. Here she explains the nature of their relationship.

> I had a boyfriend and this boyfriend used to be so abusive with me. He had other girlfriends also, but I was, oh . . . the way I was with him, I liked him a lot. I was . . . even with him when I liked him a lot . . . on a Saturday mornings I don't have any money—we spent all our money. 'Cause he don't work, I was only working—he didn't. All my money's out. I don't have food in my house.

In this instance, Elaine specifically cites infidelity as a form of abuse that she had to endure, and it was the price she had to pay to maintain the relationship with her boyfriend at the time. Without her consent, this same man disclosed her HIV status to other women in her block of flats, which led to a great deal of stigmatization of her in the neighborhood. Elaine also alludes to his having forced her to have sex in this section of the interview.

> But he was very nice when he was sober, but when he's drunk . . . He used to . . . he wasn't so . . . with me he wasn't violent, but he just want to have sex. That's all he want. He wasn't violent and he likes to drink. If I haven't got money, then I don't see him. But when I got money, then I see him. He was like that.

Elaine, like Priscilla, stops short of accusing her ex-boyfriend of raping her, but what she describes appears to be repeated coercive sex bordering on rape if not fitting the standard legal definition. The ability of women to name the abuse they have experienced may be linked to public awareness of the issue of gender-based violence (Boonzaier, 2001). The forms in which gender-based violence are experienced may not only be the forms that are most widely publicized. Thus, women may not identify an instance of abuse as true abuse, simply because it was not "violent enough." In addition to Elaine's boyfriend "just wanting to have sex," it seems he has also perpetrated acts of economic violence against her. In many instances, economic abuse results from a woman's economic dependency on men (Hoosen & Collins, 2004), which gives the men leverage and control in a relationship. In Elaine's case, her boyfriend was spending all of her money that may have otherwise gone toward her and her children's needs. It seems that Elaine carried on in this relationship in order to keep her partner in her life, which may have been a much-needed source of normalcy for her.

Elaine now has a new partner whom she claims is supportive and caring and even sympathetic to her feelings about her old boyfriend. She and her current partner heard about an accident that her ex-boyfriend was in, and she talked about her visit to see him after his accident.

> Me and my boyfriend that I have now was there by him last week. Here in the holidays we went to him—he had an accident . . . I was there by him in the

hospital. It was a car accident here on Grand Road. But he had a hole here in his head. His neck was broken in three parts. He's now so thin. I said to my boyfriend, "He's so thin. He's not that person he used to be." He used to shave nice clean. Head is clean. Nice clean clothes on. But now he stink. He's brown, brown, brown. I said, "You know what, when we come back again we gonna buy you some stuff. Shaving stuff and soap." Because now he's staying with his mother, and he said his mother is the only person that work and he get disability [social grant]. I say, "What you doing with your disability? But we gonna buy you shaving stuff, soap, toothbrush, and toothpaste and you must clean yourself . . . You aren't that person you used to be."

Now that he is in a desperate situation, Elaine has sympathy for her ex-boyfriend and has decided to care for him, even though he used to spend all of her money and, possibly, abused her sexually.

Intimate Partner Violence

In addition to being a problem for women who are already HIV positive, violence against women is an important factor in women's becoming infected with HIV. Gender-based violence and sexual power issues are increasingly being recognized as reasons for the rising incidence of HIV infection in women around the globe. Women in South Africa between the ages of 15 and 29 have the highest prevalence of HIV (Kistner, 2003). This same demographic group has the highest incidence of abuse by a partner. Kim (2002) describes these findings as "extremely significant because they indicate that young women, the demographic group which is already at higher risk of HIV infection in South Africa, simultaneously represent precisely the group which is at highest risk of rape" (p. 9).

The link between HIV and gender-based violence has been identified in the literature only since about the turn of the century, although there were hints of reference to it before 2000. Since then, research has shown a direct link. For example, a study conducted in Brazil found that women who were survivors of gender-based violence were less likely to use condoms because of gender inequalities that decreased their autonomy (Chacham, Maia, Greco, Silva & Greco, 2007). Other studies conducted in South Africa, like the ones by Kalichman and Simbayi (2004) and Dunkle and her colleagues (2004), acknowledge this link but point out that it is under-researched. Finally, in a new report from UN Women (2012), the two issues are presented as being clearly linked: "Violence against women and HIV/AIDS are . . . inextricably intertwined and mutually reinforcing in the lives of millions of women and girls: women who are subject to violence are more likely to contract HIV than other women, and women who are HIV-positive face a heightened risk of violence" (p. 1). However, this same report goes on to explain that at the program and policy level, violence against women and HIV are still being dealt with as separate problems.

"Gender-based violence" is a broad term used to describe perpetration of any type of harm against individuals based on gender (Csaky, 2008) and encompasses other, more specific terms such as "violence against women" and "intimate partner violence"; sometimes the three terms are used interchangeably. Gender-based violence is defined in detail in Kistner's (2003) literature review for the South African Department of Health as "violence directed against a person on the basis of his or her gender identity" (p. 12). This type of violence has been described as "one of the most obvious ways to convey the power difference between women and men" (Kurz, 2001, p. 205). Most people think of gender-based violence as limited to rape or the ambiguous legal term "sexual assault." Violence against women, however, takes many forms. Kistner (2003, p. 28) lists the following examples of gender-based violence: rape; battery; sexual abuse of girls; female genital mutilation; dowry-related violence; domestic violence, including marital rape; intimate femicide; non-spousal violence; violence related to exploitation; sexual harassment or intimidation at work or school; trafficking women and girls or forced prostitution; violence perpetrated by the state; secondary victimization/humiliation at the hands of police or healthcare workers; and economic violence, including the withholding of money. Gender-based violence and the potential fear thereof have a marked impact on many aspects of women's lives.

Gender-based violence is often not reported; therefore, most scholars believe that the small proportion of acts that are reported represent much larger real numbers. Large-scale surveys of the prevalence of gender-based violence are conducted in many countries, but their findings may be misleading because of underreporting. In a report for the UN Division for the Advancement of Women, Kishor (2005) cautions us in our use and understandings of large-scale prevalence survey data. Kishor points out that with surveys there is no face-to-face contact with women, and they are not given a second opportunity to report violence. The data are not very in-depth and were collected at a single point in time as opposed to those studies that use more longitudinal data-collection methods that would give women the chance to become more familiar with the research in which they are taking part, therefore increasing the likelihood that they would disclose instances of violence. In addition to the fact that non-reporting and underreporting of gender-based violence is in part due to "the culture of silence around the topic of domestic violence" (p. 7), it is also likely due to the threat of violence as a result of reporting or disclosing the violence. For example, the fact that the National Woman Abuse Action Project (Kurz, 2001) reports that battering is the most common cause of injury to women in the United States illustrates just how large that number may actually be. The hidden rates of violence against women have also been reported in many other nations.

Not only is violence against women prevalent, but it also is highly damaging. A significant proportion of women who are battered are seriously injured and must seek medical attention (Novello, 1992). Gender-based violence creates great costs to the individuals who are battered, and it is also costly for society as a whole. One particular result of violence against women that winds up being especially expensive to both the woman survivor as well as society is HIV infection. According to Raj, Silverman, and Amaro (2004), men who abuse women are more likely to engage in behaviors that put them at a greater risk for HIV infection. Many times these same men end up infecting their female partners through acts of overt or covert violence.

Linking Gender-Based Violence and HIV

There are several ways that the literature describes women's vulnerability to gender-based violence and a possible subsequent HIV infection: (1) some women are raped, and as a result of the actual physical trauma they are more vulnerable to HIV infection (Kistner, 2003); (2) violence or threats might inhibit a woman's ability to negotiate condom use within an intimate heterosexual relationship (Guedes, 2004); (3) sexual abuse in childhood could lead to riskier behaviors in adulthood (Kistner, 2003); (4) disclosure of HIV status to a partner may result in violence (Rothenberg, 1995; Seidel & Ntuli, 1996; Temmerman, 1995; Van der Straten, King, Grinstead, Serufilira & Allen, 1995); and (5) those who are abused may find themselves in desperate situations forcing them into sex work to support themselves (Dunkle et al., 2004) or leading them to resort to illegal drug use (often needle drugs) to numb themselves, exposing them to HIV. In addition, these activities expose women to other health problems (such as STIs) that can make them more easily infected by HIV or can exacerbate other illnesses if they are already infected by HIV (Kalichman & Simbayi, 2004). Thus, the research shows us that there is a strong link between women's experiences of gender-based violence and potential HIV infection.

Violence may also prevent women from obtaining treatment once they have become infected. Although there is little literature on the impact of violent events on women who are enrolled in antiretroviral (ARV) programs, it is reasonable to assume that there is some sort of impact on adherence to these medications. This assumption is strengthened by the fact that receiving a positive HIV test result is reason enough to cause posttraumatic stress disorder (PTSD), which has been shown to negatively affect adherence to ARVs (Brief et al., 2004) as well as affect the functioning of a person's already-jeopardized immune system (Delahanty, Bogart & Figler, 2004). In a meta-analysis of ninety-five studies on the relationship between depression and ARV adherence, Gonzalez and his colleagues (2011) found that the "relationship between depression and HIV treatment nonadherence is consistent across samples and over time" (p. 181) and that depression is likely a comorbid condition with other psychological problems such as PTSD. If a woman who receives a positive HIV test is also being victimized by interpersonal violence, she is undoubtedly even more vulnerable to PTSD or depression and is therefore likely to have difficulty adhering to the ARV regimens. But research on the specifics of these interactions is not yet available. Although gender-based violence has been linked to HIV infection for women, both of these problems remain significant among large numbers of women, and the number of infections among women continues to grow.

Dilemmas in the Ethics of Care

Remarkably, some of the HIV-positive women we interviewed disregard the problem of violent men because they feel that caring for men is, in part, a passport into normalcy, even when the men for whom they are caring are abusive and a financial burden. This is exacerbated in the specific context of South Africa, where men are often chronically unemployed and women are frequently the sole breadwinners of a partnership (Boonzaier, 2005). Boonzaier and de la Rey (2004) found that because of this "gender reversal," men claim to feel emasculated. Some men in their study express their frustration with their inability to carry out their proper gender expectations, which they say leads to instances of violence against their women partners. This gender reversal may also affect women's view of themselves. One way of explaining why the women we interviewed stay in non-beneficial or even abusive relationships is that the women need men as a gender prop, so to speak—meaning, women need men to maintain the veneer of normalcy for themselves as well as society, so they must often settle for and take care of men who are less than supportive, caring partners.

But are the women revealing a weakness in caring for the men they perceive as their partners, as humans in need of care, and as community members similarly stigmatized as themselves by their HIV status? Or are their values and actions ones to emulate? This dilemma in the ethics of care is at the heart of our understanding of women and their caregiving work.

Fisher and Tronto (1990) write: "On the most general level, we suggest that caring be viewed as a species activity that includes everything that we do to maintain, continue, and repair our 'world' so that we can live in it as well as possible. That world includes our bodies, our selves, and our environment, all of which we seek to interweave in a complex, life-sustaining web" (p. 103). This apparently straightforward definition presents care work as noble and as an essential feature of our humanity. In the lives of the women we interviewed, however, care work is filled with complexity. Their care work is laudable in some ways but fraught with contradictions. Their need to care for themselves and their children is intermingled with their desire to care for the men in their lives, especially when those men are HIV positive.

Marilyn Frye (1990), warns that ethics are constructed by those in power and that what we may consider to be the "right thing to do" may actually reinforce oppressive structures. Frye (2010) writes: "Sensitivity is one of the few virtues that has been assigned to us [women]. If we are found insensitive, we may fear we have no redeeming traits at all and perhaps are not real women. Thus are we silenced before we begin: the name of our situation drained of meaning and our guilt mechanisms tripped." And we see this side of the women's dilemma as well. Their care work in fact does reinforce/support oppressive relationships between themselves and the men in their lives; in doing so it negates their need to care for themselves or to create new approaches that challenge the structures in which that oppression is embedded.

Fisher and Tronto (1990) conclude that the key to understanding these issues is to view the context of care. They write: "In order to reshape caring activities, we ultimately need to reenvision social institutions. The women's movement of this generation has made very important contributions to this process. To build a feminist future we need to stretch our imaginations so that we can discover new visions of society in which caring is a central value and institutions truly facilitate real caring" (p. 56). The women in our study outlined some of the essential considerations that will need to be addressed in our reenvisioning and rebuilding.

9 Women's Bodies

> Throughout history, ideas about the nature of women's bodies have played a dramatic role in either challenging or reinforcing power relationships between women and men. As such, we can regard these ideas as political tools and can regard the struggle over these ideas as a political struggle.
>
> Rose Weitz, *The Politics of Women's Bodies*

CLASHES OVER WHAT women's bodies should do and what they should look like continue. Despite strides forward in women's rights on many fronts, bodies remain a persistent battleground. Some feminists even argue that as the feminist movement has grown, we are moving backward on issues related to women's bodies, asserting that a backlash has developed that seeks to reinforce ever more policing and regulation, including increasingly restrictive ideas and actions determined to keep women's bodies and women in "their place" (Faludi, 2006). Today this backlash takes many forms, "including 1) increasing pressure on women to control the shape of their bodies; 2) attempts to define premenstrual and post-menopausal women as ill, and; 3) the rise of the anti-abortion and 'fetal rights' movements" (Weitz, 2010, p. 9).

Women who are HIV positive find themselves in the midst of these debates. Their bodies are altered by the virus itself, which causes loss of body mass as well as other visible problems, such as skin diseases. In addition, ARVs, which have been identified as perhaps our best bet for keeping HIV-positive people healthy and eventually containing and eliminating HIV, also alter human bodies in obvious ways. The stigma of HIV is thus intensified by the effects of the ARVs that we hope can save lives.

Compliance with an ARV regimen is a challenge for many reasons, and the consequences of non-adherence are dire. The nature of ARV drugs is such that by missing one or two doses, the virus will likely become resistant, compromising physical health and ultimately causing death (Wilson, Naidoo, Bekker, Cotton & Maartens, 2004). It is also important to bear in mind the nature of the virus that these ARV drugs are attempting to combat. HIV causes severely impaired immunity. It is of great import for people living with the virus to facilitate the immunity that they still have. They must be careful to avoid situations that might promote infection by other microbes or stress-induced illnesses, as well as reinfection with other strains of the ever-mutating HI virus. ARV drug treatment requires strict adherence to a rigorous drug regimen to address all of these problems.

In administering ARVs, therefore, careful attention must be paid to social context and psychological states in order to determine how the demands of the drug regimens are being supported or compromised. For those who are concerned that their physical appearance will be disfigured, adhering to or even commencing ARV treatment becomes problematic. Women are particularly vulnerable to this problem because of the gendered nature of the pressure to conform to specific beauty and body ideals.

Nowadays, with proper care and the use of ARVs, if they are available, HIV can be treated as a chronic illness. Nevertheless, the virus is still portrayed in a frightening way by the medical community and especially by the media. Health-care workers, the community, and the media still refer to this virus as AIDS, a word associated with an image of an emaciated person dying in a hospital bed (Whittaker, 1992). In addition, because of the lack of access to treatment or ignorance about seeking treatment, being HIV positive for many is not a chronic condition and the terrifying images presented by the media are not far from the truth. In South Africa, as well as in many other countries, people are visibly dying from HIV, and the media and medical establishment have publicized and emphasized these visual images. For women, the images are perhaps even more disheartening, because the ARV drugs that make HIV a chronic illness can cause changes in body shape that are not in tune with conventional ideas about feminine beauty.

ARVs Change Bodies and Body Image

Even if a person is able to overcome the many obstacles to successfully obtaining and using ARVs, she faces the added problem of bodily changes that take place from receiving ARVs, especially HAART (highly active antiretroviral therapy, which refers to using combinations of drugs to treat HIV). ARVs are medications that improve the physical (and often the emotional) health of people living with HIV, but they are frequently accompanied by severe side effects. In addition to side effects common to other drug therapies, such as nausea and dizziness, there are other noticeable effects caused by ARVs. People who are ill as a result of HIV often lose weight because of AIDS-related wasting syndrome (Wilson et al., 2004). Once some people are on ARVs, they notice their thinness is replaced by a body-shape change referred to as lipodystrophy (Persson, 2005). Lipodystrophy is a condition in which fat is gained and redistributed to a person's midsection and upper back while their face remains thin, almost gaunt. This side effect can be long-term, and it renders a person's HIV status visible. In addition to the psychological effects of a rapid and dramatic body-shape change, people on ARVs risk the stress resulting from the exposure of their HIV status because of these visible changes.

A number of studies on the psychological effects of body-shape change have been conducted with HIV-positive gay men in the Global North. These studies have shown that changes in body shape lead to negative psychological consequences in that men feel unattractive. The men also assert that the changes in their body shape reveal their HIV status, thus resulting in their being stigmatized (Persson, 2005; Sharma et al., 2007). In many cultures body-shape changes may be even more difficult for women, because in order to be seen as attractive or even normal, femininity requires women to adhere to an even narrower range of body types than are men. These kinds of body image standards are not consistent across different cultures; however, in all cultures requirements exist as to women's appearance, and the ideal images are inconsistent with women living with HIV, especially if they are on ARVs.

Only a few studies have been conducted on HIV and body image or ARVs and body image, and the research that has been conducted sometimes comes to dubious conclusions (Reynolds, Neidig, Wu, Gifford & Holmes, 2006; Collins et al., 2006). In a study done in South Africa, for example, Hurley and her colleagues (2011) found that excessive weight gain may be a problem for women and men taking ARVs because of both stigma and "cultural norms" regarding HIV and weight, and that there is therefore a "need for a greater emphasis on lifestyle and dietary counseling" (p. 650). The narrow definitions of beauty for women and their link to particular shapes and sizes of bodies suggest that this advice would be problematic for women. The study does not address the social constraints placed on women in terms of their appearance. It also fails to take into account the way in which gender shapes and exacerbates this distress. Furthermore, the research does not address the complexity of body image and beauty standards of women in the Global South and simply refers to this as "perceptions regarding weight that are applicable in the existing local cultural context" (p. 650). Even though the research may be looking at legitimate issues surrounding the links between ARVs and ideologies about bodies, it is difficult to determine which body shapes for women in southern Africa pose problems and which do not, because standards and ideals that may be valued in the South come from local as well as international sources. Nevertheless, the research does address the fact that women's bodies are under constant scrutiny, whether they are ill or not, and because AIDS is constructed as a disease that signifies the end of being beautiful for women (Harrington, 1997), this has to be taken into account in the assessment of how women living with HIV experience and see their bodies and their lives.

Body and Beauty Standards

Women all over the world are confronted with the problem of body image and standards of beauty. In the Global South these problems are confounded by contradictory measures across different cultures; little research has been conducted on exactly what comprises these varying aesthetics and how they differ from one culture to the next. Furthermore, racism is added to the mix when ideals of feminine beauty are associated with images of tall, thin, blue-eyed blondes. Body image and beauty standards for Coloured women in South Africa are affected by all of these layers of complexity. One of the roots of the standards for South African women emerged from the cultural mix, tensions, and oppression of long years of slavery, colonialism, and apartheid in South Africa. White European colonial slaveholders' beauty standards were valued in much the same way as they are today, as well as in the rest of the world. In addition, historically, South African women's bodies were scrutinized and analyzed, part by part, under the lens of racist European colonists and their sets of standards. One of the most infamous examples of this is exemplified in the story of Saartjie Baartman.

Saartjie Baartman was a Khoisan woman from South Africa who in 1810 was taken from her home to Europe by British colonists. Baartman was swindled and coerced into traveling the world with her exploiters to display her body to white Westerners. European voyeurs dissected and exploited her body in attempts to defend racist assumptions and to sexualize African women (Wiss, 1994). As well, she became a visual fascination for white Europeans, because they believed she did not resemble them or their ideals of white beauty. Baartman was forced to perform naked at public events in Europe. After her death, her labia and brain were preserved and a plaster cast was made of her body and displayed until the 1970s in France. In 2002 Nelson Mandela was able to bring her remains back to South Africa, and she was finally buried in Gamtoos Valley. South African women's bodies have a history of being othered for reasons of race and nationality, and today the othering process is compounded by disease.

Beauty, Bodies, HIV, and South African Women Today

The discourse of expectations about beauty and women's bodies emerged as a significant one in our study. The women talked about their bodies and their beauty in four main ways: (1) how they used to look before finding out they are living with HIV; (2) how the illness has made them and HIV-positive people in the media look; (3) how ARVs make them and others taking the medications look; and (4) how they think ARVs will make them look if they decide to commence treatment.

When asked about how their lives have changed since receiving a positive HIV test, the women we interviewed talked about what they looked like before they were tested for HIV. Priscilla talked about how her daily struggles for food and money have been magnified since she found out she is living with HIV. She reminisced about the days when she still had time for herself.

> I totally changed, Anna. I totally changed, honestly. And you know, I don't even have time for myself. You know? Before I found out I'm HIV, I was

always . . . how can I say? . . . If your hair is beautiful, then your face is also beautiful. My hair was always rolled in, you know. I was always looking after myself. But the moment I found out, I lost totally control. I'm not the same person.

When she uses phrases such as "I totally changed" and "I'm not the same person" in reference to her physical beauty, Priscilla suggests she is not who she once was and is not as good as she once was. Her words allude to her feeling that because her appearance has changed, her entire person has been altered or damaged. This suggestion is startling, because at the time of the interview, Priscilla had known of her positive status for less than two years.

Priscilla went on to speak about having mixed feelings when people pay her compliments on the way she looks. She told us about returning to the neighborhood she used to live in and the reactions of the people there seeing her for the first time in a long time. Her former neighbors were excited to see her again and complimented her on her appearance. Priscilla wants to feel good about being complimented and welcomed after so long, but she also described the painful feelings that have arisen from her harboring the secret of living with HIV, and in some ways she feels unworthy of the compliments.

> But to tell the truth, Anna, that is what I think of myself. I'm not that person anymore, and I don't look cute or whatever. But when I go to people that they don't see me for a long time, they always tell me, "Ooh, you are just the same. You are cute! You got a *lekker* [nice] figure." You know—so. I can't believe that the people said I look so cute and so sexy. You know, I will think a lot of bad things about me because I'm HIV.

Here again, Priscilla uses the phrase "I'm not that person anymore" in reference to her physical appearance. But her words signify something more, because at the end of the excerpt she says that she "think[s] a lot of bad things about me because I'm HIV," which tell us how unworthy she feels about the compliments. Not only has she lost what she used to be, but also she believes she is now an unworthy, "bad" person.

Linda, too, talked about how her body used to look before she initially lost weight and the subsequent change in body shape she experienced because of the ARVs.

> Because I used to wear size 36 [approximately U.S. size 10] . . . those flair skirts I never wear now anymore, because I don't have hips anymore, I don't have bums anymore [laughing]! . . . I can wear other clothes. I've got clothes that I didn't wear anymore . . . You know, the next meeting I'll bring you my pictures that I took when I was size 36.

In the above excerpt, Linda points out that she does not "have hips" and does not "have bums" because of the side effects from ARVs. Her words suggest a disconnection or a focus on the individual parts of her body that she is not happy with or that have changed. This type of dismemberment is reminiscent of the objectification and commodification of women's bodies found in Western advertising media and pornography (Kirk & Okazawa-Rey, 2004).

As part of her response to the question about what the biggest changes in her life have been since being diagnosed as HIV positive, Elvyra spoke about how she used to look. She explained how she used to be involved in several different sports and how her diagnosis led her to become depressed and to cease involvement in athletic activities.

> ELVYRA: I played badminton and all that. Yeah! I was a 60 [kilograms, or about 132 pounds]; my weight was 65 . . . 68. Yeah. Yeah. And badminton. I played badminton.
>
> ANNA: Why did you stop . . . being athletic after . . .
>
> ELVYRA: Because I felt very disappointed. Because you don't feel active anymore.

The mention of her weight is significant here, because Elvyra is now quite thin. A weight of 60–68 kilograms is significantly more than she weighs now. She expresses her disappointment that her athleticism has waned. In addition to describing her weight changes, Elvyra is also suggesting that her body is no longer strong, agile, and athletic as it once was.

Body Size Rules and Regulations

Although the women we interviewed spoke about beauty ideals and maintaining their beauty in ways that are generally the same as we might find among women in the North, the specifics of their concerns about body size and weight were quite different. The North, perhaps most significantly the United States, is arguably the source of some of the most stringent and enduring, thus hegemonic, body and beauty standards for women. Women in the Global North are expected to uphold a certain set of extreme physical characteristics (Kirk & Okazawa-Rey, 2004) in order to gain entry into society and access to men in particular. Increasingly women are resorting to surgical procedures as the only way to attain the standards. More than 9 million cosmetic surgical procedures at a cost of nearly $10 billion were performed in the United States in 2011. The top five in order were liposuction, breast augmentation, tummy tucks, eyelid surgery, and breast lifts (Mann, 2012).

One of the most prominent features of the sets of standards reflected in these surgical procedures is the necessity of having a body that is as thin as can be. In the North a woman's thin, specifically proportioned body is a mark of her morality and her will to exert self-control (Bordo, 1993). In addition to signifying her drive for success and mastery over her body, the necessity of thinness draws on the increasing biomedical discourse surrounding the array of purported health risks associated with obesity (Huff, 2001). The ways in which the women in our study spoke about their concerns over their loss of weight due to medical problems or stress, however, reflect a different set of standards. They were concerned that they have lost their sexy bodies because they have become so thin. Similarly, in research with women in rural Jamaica, Sobo (1994) points out that the bigger a woman's body is, the more beautiful and healthy she is considered. The women in our study explained that they feel the need to appear weighty enough so that they do not look unhealthy. In addition, they described their previous heavier bodies as more beautiful and capable—for example, in playing sports.

It could be said that the very notion that women must appear in a particular way is a Northern one, but it is difficult to say whether the Northern expectations of thinness in women are a more oppressive ideal than the ideal of a larger body among rural women in Jamaica. In any event, women in both places are compelled to appear in a certain way. It seems that expectations in the North, however, are more rigid and widespread and the consequences more significant. The message is a powerful one, and increasingly these Western beauty standards and expectations of women are becoming more common for women globally (Kirk & Okazawa-Rey, 2004), specifically in the Global South. Images of beauty and body ideals are disseminated throughout the globe in the form of media that are largely produced in the Global North, so the rest of the world sees and processes the images and incorporates them into their own cultures (Zeleza, 2002, July, as cited in Salo, 2005). The media industry in the United States as well as Bollywood from India (which reflects many of the same components of Northern beauty ideals) and the media images of beauty these institutions pump into South Africa cannot be ignored by women. Other studies in South Africa reflect similar findings, where women interviewed speak about fatness connoting dignity and strength while at the same time saying it is desirable to be thin (see, for example, Puoane, Fourie, Shapiro, Tshaka & Oelefse, 2005; Puoane, Tsolekile & Steyn, 2010). These beauty ideas fuel gender-stratified, capitalist societies in that women are compelled to consume a variety of goods and services that facilitate these ideals (and if they cannot, they are marginalized further), which simultaneously support capitalism and maintain the oppression of women (Kirk & Okazawa-Rey, 2004).

Looking Like "AIDS"

The women we interviewed are keenly aware of how people living with HIV are portrayed on TV and in other media. The women talked about the physical appearance of HIV-positive people on TV and how those images have affected how they see themselves and the decisions they must make to contend with HIV.

Tisha was asked how she came to the decision to take ARVs. She spoke about how she needed treatment because she was physically ill, but what ultimately motivated her to make the decision was the images she witnessed on TV.

> I had to take the tablet for my . . . see, because I was sick, *ne* [you know]? And then I heard and saw people on TV, saw people in newspaper who are dying of AIDS, and then I was scared that maybe to happen to me, and then I started to . . . to take my treatment.

In Tisha's case physical health alone was not enough to motivate her to take treatment for HIV; when her physical appearance was called into play, however, she says she was more willing to take the risk of commencing ARV treatment.

Elaine also talked about her fear of looking like "the people on TV." Elaine admitted that sometimes she questions whether she really is HIV positive, because she doesn't resemble the images of AIDS in the media.

> Sometimes I feel in my mind, "Are you really HIV positive?" Because I feel like a . . . if I see the people on TV . . . then I say to myself, "Ohhh, are you going to look like that?" . . . And they say it put sores on their mouth and tongue and all that. And I thought to myself, "Elaine, you never had that stuff. The only thing you got is shingles, but you never had sores in your mouth." Something like that. They say it's a death penalty.

The notion of "AIDS as a death penalty" and the graphic images perpetuated in the media are also part of a discourse of fear of the virus and people who are living with it. The ideas and images of people who are visibly ill probably have a great deal to do with why the women we interviewed frequently spoke of their physical appearance since their diagnosis.

The media have portrayed HIV with shocking visuals. It is not difficult to find images of people in advanced stages of AIDS, their bodies extremely thin or covered with lesions. The imagery around HIV is unique in this way. It is possible, for example, to access online images of people living with any disease, but HIV is disproportionately represented visually and the images available are especially shocking and graphic. Why the media present images of HIV in this way is a question with no definitive answer. On the one hand, some of the images are designed to scare people into getting tested, which could benefit those who are tested or the public health in general (although this benefit will not be realized by those who do not have access to health care). It may also be the case that the media are sensationalizing the pandemic as a way to increase their own revenues. The shocking nature of the images may also serve as a way of othering those who are HIV positive, shifting the blame of the pandemic from those of us who are "normal and healthy" to those who are "deviant" or who have done something to "deserve" HIV infection. Either way, large media sources have generated a frightening visual story of HIV and AIDS.

The media, of course, have for many years generated the visual story of women. A woman's body is something that has been made into an object that can be identified as beautiful or ugly, fat or thin, normal or abnormal, acceptable or unacceptable, white or black, and healthy or unhealthy. In the context of South Africa, where food is scarce and many of the women we interviewed speak frequently of food or lack thereof, body weight and appearance take on an added dimension. With the knowledge of their positive HIV status, the women with whom we spoke suddenly became very aware of weight fluctuations. They ask "Am I too thin?" and "Do I look like I have AIDS now?" Their thinness reveals their poverty and suggests that they might not be healthy. In addition, it may indicate that they are HIV positive. In Cape Town people often talk about whether people have lost or gained weight. But in contrast to the concerns about weight that people in the United States might have, especially for weight gain, Capetonians speak about someone's weight loss as a problem or an indication that something stressful is happening in their life or that they may be using drugs. People are positive in talking about weight gain because it is usually an indication that the person is being taken care of by a spouse and that they are happy. Weight gain in Cape Town is associated with such factors as getting married and being contented or having a job that affords food, especially meat on the table every day.

Making the Decision to Take ARVs

While the distress the women feel about their changing appearance resulting from HIV is emotionally painful and may exacerbate their physical problems, ironically it can also serve as a motivation for seeking ARVs that will help them to feel better and to live longer. At one point in our interview with Elaine, she explained why she finally decided to take ARVs.

> Yes, and through the *dingis* [translates to thing, but here she means goodness] of God that I'm still . . . and through the ARVs that I'm using that keep me going. 'Cause I was very, very thin. I was so afraid to go out of the house. I was thin, thin, thin. And then afterwards, I go on the ARVs. The doctor asked me do I want to go on the ARVs. I'm now on these ARVs for three years. Now the doctor asked me, "Do you want to go on ARVs?" I said, "Yes, doctor."

In the above excerpt, Elaine explains that because she was "very, very thin," she felt compelled to commence ARV therapy. The word "thin" connotes appearance, and it is in fact the only physical issue she points to as the driving force behind the commencement of ARV therapy. She does not mention discomfort, weakness, or specific health difficulties as a reason for starting ARVs. Elaine's words suggest she started the treatment primarily because of her appearance, yet this is not entirely a question of vanity. She says that her thinness indicates that she is getting sicker, so she accepted the doctor's suggestion to begin ARVs. But the way she describes her thinking behind this decision reveals that she is concerned with how HIV is making her thin and that others can see that "something is wrong"—in particular, that they may discover she is living with HIV.

Linda also talked about how her worries about losing weight and the thin appearance of her body are a result of stress. She had been staying with her sister and brother-in-law until he became abusive and forced Linda to leave. Here she talks about a discussion she had with her employer and how the eviction made her feel.

> It really makes me feel very down, you know. And I lose a lot of weight because I was stressing. Yeah. So they were so worried, and so they just tell me, "You know that you don't . . . you shouldn't be stressed." I said, "How can I control the stress? I can't control the stress." So now I lose weight.

In fact, Linda's employers also seem to be becoming obsessed with monitoring the appearance of her body and weight. Linda claims to feel both appreciative of this and bothered by it at the same time. She told us about a conversation she had with her employer in which he discussed her weight.

> "You must try and eat this. If you want your weight." So every day they say to me maybe once or twice . . . there is a scale [laughing] . . . they showed me how to work the scale . . . they said, "We'll monitor your weight now [laughing]." They said, "Yeah, we'll take care of you," you know? I said, "Yeah . . . I appreciate it but . . ." sometimes they can talk things that makes me feel stressed out, you know? Sometimes I think, "If I could go—leave them."

Linda struggles to maintain a particular weight that she finds suitable for her health as well as her appearance. But she experiences the constant monitoring of her weight by herself and her employers as an intrusion and an added source of anxiety as well.

Priscilla also has disturbing thoughts about her body because she feels she is getting thinner. She explained that she has been unable to find work, and this leaves her with too much time to think about the fact that she is HIV positive.

> If my mind just flows . . . I'm just, "Oh, I'm HIV . . . I'm so thin." My pants, my panties all fall. So that's why I must go look for something that keeps me busy, Anna.

It is significant that Priscilla explains that if her mind is not occupied, she first thinks of her positive HIV status, and only second to that worry is her body image being "so thin."

She spoke again about compliments she has received that she can no longer accept because of how she now sees herself as an embodiment of the HI virus.

> When I go to my brother [in another neighborhood], then his friends would always tell me, "You look beautiful! Still young!" You know—so. "You would never say you got four kids." And I feel so proud, I can't believe it. Honestly. Then I ask them, "Really?" "You are sexy. *Yoh* [meaning wow]! You got four

kids, your eldest daughter is 15 . . . You look nice after you." I can't believe it, because I didn't think that of myself. When I look in the mirror, then I told myself, "You're not that Priscilla anymore . . ." You know? That is what I said. But I mustn't do that to myself. I mustn't. Every morning when I look in the mirror, I must always say, "Thank you, God . . . beautiful girl and . . ." You know? But to tell the truth, Anna, that is [not] what I think of myself. I'm not that person anymore and I don't look cute or whatever.

Priscilla's perception of her appearance since her HIV test has deteriorated, even though others apparently do not see these changes. They continue to see her as attractive, but she has internalized her negative feelings. Maybe Priscilla has not changed on the outside, but her mind has changed. She has internalized HIV stigma and punishes herself with her thoughts even though those in her immediate circle do not share her point of view.

This idea that Priscilla's thinness is connected to her HIV and indicates there is something wrong with her, however, is not just something she is telling herself. Her partner has reminded her that her thinness is not only a sign that she is HIV positive; it is also a sign that she may have infected him. He talks about Priscilla's appearance as it relates to HIV. She relayed to us an argument she frequently has with her partner about how he became infected and subsequently infected her.

So, Anna, he told me, "Before I came to you," he did have someone but not a steady girlfriend, just a "hit-and-run." So he told me, "Maybe Priscilla, she gave it to me." That was his words to me. But out of the blue he told me, "No, it cannot be she, because she's fat. And this illness is something that makes you thin." He told me, "You are thin, Priscilla, but she is fat. No, I don't think she gave it to me." So I don't know, Anna. For me, it is so confused, you know?

Priscilla's negative feelings about her appearance are not just related to her size. She also talked about changes she has seen in her skin. She told us the changes took place over the past few weeks.

Anna, I know myself, I know my body, I know my skin. You know? This is still the second week that I see my hands is not the same. My skin, it looks darker, and my face is also getting darker, because my sister told me, "Oh, your skin is getting black now and a lot of pimples coming on your face." So I told her, "Oh, well . . . I'm getting old now." But you know, it's the second week that I see my hands. My hands are very thin and my skin is not the same. It feels so . . . I cannot even tell you, but my skin looks like a tortoise. My skin looks like that. Honestly. You cannot see it, Anna, because you will not understand, you will not know . . . you know, but I know my skin, I know myself. It's totally different.

As she spoke, Priscilla looked down at her hands with an expression of disgust as if she could hardly stand her own appearance and literally did not want to be in her own skin. Although she looked fine to us during the interview, she expressed a lot of self-loathing. In these comments, Priscilla speaks again of her appearance in how her hands and skin are "not the same"; in fact, they are "totally different." She uses this kind of language throughout her descriptions of the visible physical changes she believes have taken place since testing positive, suggesting that there have been drastic changes in her appearance.

Since Priscilla has tested positive for HIV, she and her partner have become hyperaware of her appearance in comparison to other perceived "healthy" people. The hyperawareness is reflected in her language too—"it's not the same," "you cannot see it," "it's totally different." Because Priscilla believes she has been living with the virus for only one or two years and she claims to have a relatively high CD4 count, it is not clear if her weight loss and skin changes are due to the physiological effects of the virus or her psychological decline. Still she sees her appearance as a measure of her health in regard to HIV. This is problematic, because today the experience of HIV is immersed in a context that sets impossible standards for bodies, beauty, and normalcy for women. To be beautiful and normal requires that women meet many stringent standards, including not appearing to be living with HIV.

ARVs and "Womanly" Bodies

Discussions of ARVs were another issue the women we interviewed talked about in relation to their feelings about their bodies and their appearance. Some women described how ARVs have made them gain weight and look less like someone who is ill; other women talked about the negative effects the ARVs have had on their appearance; and finally, there was talk surrounding the fear of commencing ARV treatment because of what the women have seen and heard happens to one's body as a result of the medicine.

Linda had a lot to say about the effect of ARVs on a person's body. She told us about a woman who was previously in the support group whose body changed when she began taking ARVs.

> There was another lady . . . she's no longer in the group. She was thin like me. Phew! The day she come, she was bigger than you. The hips! Especially the hips, as if somebody put these steaks on the side here. But here [touching her waist] she was so thin. She was . . . Phew, she was beautiful!

Linda also talked about how her own appearance has gone through changes she says are caused by ARVs. She described some of the negative side effects.

> I didn't have those other bad side effects that cause me to sleep in hospital like other—other people they will get admitted [into the hospital]. The only thing that I did have—it loses your shaping . . . becoming . . . you lose your shape. If you like this [hourglass gesture], you see you've got a figure and hips and that.

> You becoming another thing, you know? Your bums becoming . . . if you did have big bums—they getting . . . they dropping! . . . Yes! They dropping down [laughing]. And then you've got your . . . your boobs . . . becoming big—you're becoming shapeless! I was worried about that [laughing]! I just complained about that. Because they ask you, "What do you feel now?" I said, "I'm feeling [concerned with the changes in her body] . . ." Because if they check me, "You healthy! So what is wrong?" I said no. Because also I did lose weight about that problem and I told them . . . they said, "Yeah, but you're healthy! You're not sick . . . the important thing is that you're not sick."

In these comments Linda is saying that ARVs may improve one's health, but in her case the changes she experienced in her body shape were not what she would consider an improvement.

Linda relayed to us her discussion with her children and her doctor about how the initial changes in her body as a side effect of the ARVs has caused her to actually lose weight again because of the related stress. Now the doctors, her children, and she herself are trying to convince her that her body shape is coming back to "normal" and that the important thing is that she is physically healthy.

> So all the time now when I'm wearing clothes, I can feel myself now. If I am walking, I can feel myself now—I am better. So I said to my children, "How do I look?" They say, "Mom, you fine now. Now you good." I say, "Really?" They say, "Yeah, it's not like that time." I say, "Okay [laughing]." . . . I don't know why . . . and if you complain to the doctor, they say, "We can't do anything, because, yes, they [ARVs] do this . . . it's other side effects or other . . . they do that shapelessness, but as long as you stay alive. It's what we most worried about."

Although Linda told us her health is her primary concern, she spoke at length about the negative changes she has seen in her appearance. "Health" is what she and her doctors seem to be striving for, but as Linda has said, worry about her appearance has caused her so much stress that she has lost weight at times, which indeed has an effect on her health. Fortunately, in the above excerpt, Linda seems to be coming to terms with her changed body, and perhaps she has convinced herself that worrying about her weight and body shape are not what she should focus on.

Priscilla, who is not on ARVs, mentioned several reasons for not commencing ARV treatment. One reason is the ongoing problem in South Africa as to the choice that people living with HIV must make between receiving social disability grants or receiving ARVs (Hardy & Richter, 2006). Priscilla mentioned that she needs the social disability grant that she may be eligible for when her CD4 count is low enough and when the government recognizes her as disabled. She is aware that the chances for receiving a grant will be diminished if she goes on medication. Priscilla was also concerned with commencing ARV treatment because of the physical effects they have on a person's appearance.

> I did tell you the truth . . . I don't think, like I see for myself . . . I see a lot of pills, medicine . . . it gives you side effects if you use it, and I'm scared to go on treatment like that. You know, like the doctor, he told me it's very good for, umm . . . the ARVs—he said that is a very good drug or whatever, but he told me it is very good . . . I did hear a lot what the people say it can give you side effects. You know, I did see side effects. You know, it's not nice on your legs, arms, and you know how's the people [how they will gossip about changes in her appearance] . . . But I don't know, Anna, like I told you, I'm very scared about ARVs, because I read a lot about ARVs. And I did see what did ARVs do to people, because people did tell me—this is what ARVs do. I'm really scared. To tell you the truth, I'm really scared.

So the choices, as they relate to ARVs, are not simply between sickness and health. Medication for any illness comes with side effects, but the side effects are often not visible to others. Not only must women living with HIV choose between ARVs and social disability grants, but their decisions are further confounded by what the ARVs will do to their appearance. They must also consider that their physical beauty may be at stake.

Grappling with Bodies

The women we interviewed have a variety of concerns with their bodies and their appearance. Kirk and Okazawa-Rey (2004) explain that our bodies "provide us with a living, physical basis for our identity" (p. 111), either as individuals or as a community. Specifically, the human body is the primary site for the physical enactment of the constructs of gender (Reischer & Koo, 2004). In their review of the theoretical orientations of the body in research, Reischer and Koo find that the body as a "symbol" and as an "agent" emerges as an important theme (p. 297). The idea that the body is an agent, or a tool with which a goal can be accomplished, is evident in the ways women must use their bodies and appearance as agents in society. Women in particular have a special burden placed on them when it comes to their bodies. How a woman sees herself and how she presents herself, as well as how others see her and how she believes others see her, are major issues for women in a world where they are expected to conform to hegemonic standards of beauty if they want to gain acceptance and avoid stigma and further marginalization.

The standards set today for bodies, beauty, and normalcy for women are frequently impossible to achieve, even if one is what society considers a healthy person. HIV introduces further problems. Persson (2005) has described what she refers to as the "AIDS body," which has been constructed as "ugly," "different," and immoral (p. 245). South African women are conscious of their bodies in comparison to beauty norms, and an element of the standard is that they do not appear to be HIV positive (Hoosen & Collins, 2004).

For the women in our study, there is virtually no safe place for the bodies and appearances of women living with HIV. As described earlier, the women with whom we spoke are living in extreme poverty. Most live either in public housing or in shacks built on the sand of townships. In some neighborhoods there is no electricity or indoor plumbing. People use outhouses, which are unsanitary and often close to the shacks, and they must walk to a cold-water pump to get water each day for cooking and washing over a wood fire from fuel gathered on the roadside. These same women talk of struggling to find food each day; they often have to go door to door and collect small amounts of food from the people in their neighborhood until they have enough for a small meal for the family. Despite the pressures of these life-and-death struggles, including the problem of living with HIV, the women's struggle with their appearances and what they see as their fading beauty plays a central role in their lives.

In addition to being impossible to achieve, standards of beauty vary. Thin dominates as something good to be achieved, but as is apparent from the interviews, fatter women in some social contexts and cultures can be identified as more attractive and more womanly. And on top of these complexities is the question of resistance to the standards. The women in our research grapple with the validity of all of these standards and where their bodies should stand among them. Judith Lorber and Lisa Jean Moore (2007) write: "In the social construction of women's bodies, a good touchstone is, 'Don't take anything for granted.' First there is no such thing as a 'real woman.' All women's bodies are made in conformity or resistance or inventive adaptation to social norms and expectations. Second, the lines between agency and submission to social pressures are not so clear" (p. 106).

10 Lessons for the World

FIVE DISCOURSES EMERGED in our analysis of the interview transcripts: (1) being normal through work and men; (2) disclosure for better or worse; (3) taking care of children; (4) caring for violent men; and (5) women's bodies. Sometimes these mirror the dominant discourse about HIV, sometimes they pose alternative discourses, and always they reveal the tensions and links between oppression and resistance.

Our discussions of these five topics shows the women we interviewed drawing upon common ways of talking about femininity and normalcy as a means to reconstruct themselves as humans in the face of dominant discourses, which present HIV-positive women as something less than human. All five topics share an overarching core feature of wrestling with the problem of stigma and using notions and practices of femininity to attempt to overcome stigma and appear as normal and acceptable. Within each discourse, however, we also found ambiguity, contradiction, and resistance. At the same time the women attempt to appear "normal," they also question and sometimes even challenge these constructs of what it means to be real women.

Listening to Women

Our study suggests that women living with HIV face major obstacles in their lives as they struggle against stigma and othering forces. The questions we posed in our interviews came from our reading of the literature on gender and HIV. Much of the research and discussion about HIV by health-care professionals and policy makers centers on issues such as biological problems and the challenge of finding medical solutions, policy issues regarding access to ARVs, and questions that relate to educational needs such as developing greater knowledge about condoms. These are all important topics that are part of the dominant discourse on HIV as it appears among scholars, professionals, and governmental officials. However, the women we spoke with directed the conversations toward other issues about living with HIV: maintaining relationships with men who may or may not be good partners; working for wages as a way to normalize themselves; deliberating about the disadvantages as well as the benefits of disclosing one's status to family and friends as the medical and psychological communities dictate; doing care work for men partners and children while living in abusive situations; and coping with or becoming hyperaware of body changes that are brought on as a result of HIV or ARVs.

Discourses of Normalization: Work and Men

The distorted perceptions of people who are HIV positive that permeate the media and become part of the thinking of those who are positive, as well as those who are not, make people who are HIV positive seem almost not human. Reconstituting oneself as normal and fully human becomes a critical task for people who are living with HIV. Two "tools" that the women in our study use as ways to normalize themselves are work and men. Women speak about work as a way to earn wages that can help them meet practical material needs. However, they also speak about work as a way to normalize their lives and themselves. Going to work makes them feel that they are worthy individuals taking care of themselves and contributing to their families and the community in general. This sentiment is undoubtedly felt by women in many places in the world, but it is especially characteristic of the experience of Coloured women in South Africa. And, importantly, for Coloured women in South Africa, earning a wage is also associated with being a woman. In contrast, for example, to white American women in the mid-twentieth century, where working for a paycheck was part of being masculine, Coloured women in South Africa have historically displayed their femininity by earning wages. Under the apartheid regime that existed in South Africa prior to the revolution in 1994, Coloured women, especially in the Western Cape, sometimes had an advantage over men in the labor market, because women were given preference over men when seeking employment due to the importance of the textile and garment industry in the Western Cape province and the dominance of women's labor in this sector (Salo, 2005). This placed women in many households in the situation of being the primary breadwinners, and certain types of bread-winning evolved into a behavior identified with femininity. Although nearly two decades have now passed since the collapse of the apartheid government, the remnants of this connection are still apparent in women who feel that being a paid worker or breadwinner for their household is an ideal feminine quality. Working for wages is a way to identify oneself as a real woman.

For the women in our study, working is not only a source of pride and a sign of femininity, but with the status of breadwinner also comes power. Having access to a way to earn a living and thereby supporting themselves and their households is not only a critical source of subsistence; it is also a basis of power. This is an unusual position to be in, given that these women were living under a deliberately racist patriarchy. It is a reversal of the oppressive gender hierarchies, since work and talking about work and earning money is a fundamental feature of white masculinity that has historically predominated and continues to be central in the North. For the women we interviewed, however, talking about and doing work is decidedly feminine. Fitting into acceptable constructs of femininity is a way to be normal, to be real women, and to resist dehumanizing, denormalizing, and defeminizing stigma regarding their HIV status. Earning a wage, or at least working for material goods that they and their families can use to survive, is therefore a way to establish oneself as fully human, normal, and womanly.

The strategy of using working for wages as a path for coming back to "normal," however, is not without pitfalls. In our interviews the women spoke frequently of their work lives, emphasizing the fact that they are not only carrying out tasks that make them useful and capable, but are also carrying out the normal gendered expectations prescribed for women in their community. They also gain a degree of power in doing so in attempts to destigmatize or normalize the "abnormal" situation of being HIV positive. This process, therefore, can work in favor of women living with HIV and, arguably, does so in the case of some of the women we interviewed. But this normalization strategy, in which the women emphasize an element of femininity, may not always be to their advantage. First of all, this avenue to staking a claim as normal is not always, perhaps not often, available. Finding a stable job is difficult, because unemployment rates are high and jobs are insecure. Second, the jobs women are able to find in paid employment pay low wages and give them little autonomy. Salo's (2005) study of young women (and men) in Manenberg found that renegotiating or emphasizing femininity sometimes only moves a woman from one oppressive environment or situation to another. In the case of the women with whom we spoke, finding jobs with meager pay is advantageous because it provides at least a little money, but the jobs can hardly be seen as truly empowering employees. Finally, the belief that work makes us human plays into the belief that those who are unable to find jobs or unable to keep them because of the economy, discrimination, or illness are somehow less valuable as humans. Work does not set us free, nor should it be a test of our right to be seen as fully human beings.

A second factor the women in our study identified as important to normalizing their lives is in establishing and maintaining intimate, monogamous relationships with men. Like work, however, this strategy also has its problems. Marriage is a powerful social institution that is associated with adulthood, responsibility, and normative sexuality. Therefore, being married or in a marriage-like relationship is a way of presenting oneself to the world as an acceptable upstanding citizen. Marriage, however, can also operate as an essential tool for controlling individual women and maintaining a system that oppresses women in general. Some theorists argue that marriage may be the key to maintaining gender inequality in society. On one hand, the women in our study feel they need men as a buffer against stigma. In order to appear normal and in order to have stable intimate heterosexual partners, they believe they must have a man in their life with whom they maintain a marriage or a marriage-like relationship. On the other hand, this strategy may create even more oppressive situations for women, especially when the men are abusive, as they are in a number of the relationships of the women we interviewed. Furthermore, even when these partnerships are not abusive, they can be draining if the men need care and therefore create an emotional, physical, and economic deficit in the household for which the women are responsible.

In addition to wanting to establish what they perceive to be normal intimate heterosexual relationships as a way of buffering stigma, the women talked about love. Their notions of romantic love are part of the package of "normalization," and the connections they feel with the men in their lives provide them with emotional satisfaction. But these connections also create problems, because they are accompanied by beliefs that loving relationships include sexual interactions. Furthermore, they are tied to beliefs that loving sexual arrangements are built on trust and therefore should not be encumbered by using condoms, which imply the arrangements are not deeply loving and faithful. While love should be a central feature of our understanding of HIV, the emotional components of our sexual relationships have been largely ignored. The women in our study remind us that their feelings of strong emotional ties to the men in their lives, and the ways those ties shape their ability to protect themselves from acquiring HIV or caring for themselves if they are living with HIV, are crucial to their experience. Feelings and notions of love are ever present in their relationships although the scholarly literature and the discourse of policy makers have been mostly silent about the salience of emotions.

Discourses of Disclosure

A second discourse that emerged in our interviews involves the question of disclosure. The medical community recommends—and in South Africa as well as other places the government insists—that HIV-positive people disclose their status as part of the approved protocol for receiving benefits. The women in this study spoke about how disclosing their HIV status has affected them. Some women have disclosed with good results that allowed them to gain certain forms of social support. But others struggle with disclosing because they have had to endure a great deal of stigmatization and marginalization already, and they quite literally may not be able to afford a disclosure gone wrong. Whatever the consequence of disclosure is for an individual woman, gendered stigma by others is common and powerfully felt and is often even internalized by the woman herself (Fife & Wright, 2000). It needs to be acknowledged that although in many circumstances disclosure may help people living with HIV, it can seriously hinder them in others (Klitzman et al., 2004). Furthermore, the women in our study who expressed their anxieties about the people to whom they have not yet disclosed need to be advised that their decisions about disclosure are valid regardless of whether they decide to disclose or not. Women need to be encouraged and empowered to be confident in making their own decisions about what they perceive as a safe disclosure, and their choices need to be validated. They need to be assured that leaving the decision up in the air can be a conscious, deliberate, and sometimes the best decision given the circumstances. Disclosure should be empowering, but it requires relinquishing some of the gendered ideologies that women in this situation cling to as their only means of holding together a normal life in the margins of society.

The women remind us that focusing so narrowly on individual choices and behavior are perhaps not the best, and certainly not the only, way of thinking about how to tackle the problem of HIV stigma. The struggles with disclosure described by the women in our study suggest that the disclosure dilemma should not be posed as strictly a choice between disclosing and not disclosing. The logic of their decisions about this issue points to social context as the key factor. This suggests that we should shift our focus, or at least our exclusive focus, away from encouraging individuals to disclose and toward advocating changes in the social structures that make disclosure so risky. Rather than thinking in terms of the pros and cons of disclosing, a third option should be offered: exerting pressure on the government, the media, and society in general to do away with the structures that make stigma possible. Stigma is known to be exacerbated because of raced, classed, and gendered hierarchies. Through the process of othering and marginalization, stigma is made possible. These oppressive processes and forces allow the dominant social structures to place blame on and subsequently stigmatize, discriminate, and oppress people, especially women, whom they have constructed as "high risk," or "virus vectors," mostly because of their real status as poor people of color. One way these untruths can be overcome is through mass disclosure, which would lead to greater community acceptance of people living with HIV. But we must also think about how disclosure would uncover the truths about who or what is really to blame and why stigma is possible, which would push forward real social change. The steps toward these kinds of actions have yet to be laid out, but one step may be to more rigorously train women living with HIV how to disclose their health status in different situations and make them aware of when they should and should not consider disclosing. Most importantly, women need to understand the broader impact of these disclosures on the oppressive forces in society. Through such knowledge they can decide where their personal decisions fit best into their own lives as well as into the larger social context, and they can consider the actions they and others might take to challenge the inequities and injustice in that social context.

Discourses of Care Work

A third issue we heard about from the women in our study is doing care work for men and children in their lives. The first observation we can make about this issue, of course, is the fact that the burden of caregiving is most often shouldered by women. In fact, it appears that women feel compelled to do this work because they believe it is expected of them as their feminine duty regardless of the real situation in which they find themselves. They carry on doing the work for men and children even when the men are abusive, the children are resistant, and when they themselves are in greater need of care than those for whom they are caring. The fact that some of the men in their lives are violent and continue to inflict abuse on their partners in myriad ways while benefiting from the care provided by the women they abuse also indicates that gendered expectations have gone very wrong.

The gendered hegemonic discourses women draw on in speaking of caring for their partners and children indicate the need for reshaping the hegemonic structure of femininity as well as masculinity. Although this is a lofty goal, there is a glimmer of hope in that there are now studies such as the one by Boonzaier and de la Rey (2004) in which men as well as women are involved in the exploration of violence against women. There is also now a recent trend in research and intervention with men along the lines of gender transformation and some of the programs designed to change the ways men do gender (i.e., violence against women) have proven successful (see Barker, Ricardo & Nascimento, 2007, for a comprehensive review of such programs). On a grassroots level there is talk in the international HIV activist community as well as in HIV support groups in Cape Town about directing support toward couples. The goal is to address issues such as care work and abuse with perpetrators as well as survivors of abuse. These types of strategies are hopeful, because despite the relatively more powerful position in which men are placed in comparison to women, both men and women in the community where our interviews took place are marginalized because of their ethnicity and socioeconomic status. As more people become infected with HIV and converge in support groups, there are more instances in which men as well as women can learn about sources of violence. It will become more and more apparent that when one is poor and marginalized from the rest of the world because of race ethnicity, nationality, and HIV status, reacting against the power structures makes more sense than attacking a woman partner.

The women in our study see and feel deeply about their connection, empathy, and camaraderie with the men in their lives. As outsiders we might judge them as making foolish or self-destructive decisions, but while their decisions to stay with and care for abusive men are certainly not in their individual interest, we need to listen to why they have made these decisions. The glue that holds partners together is a complex mix of gender injustice coupled with centuries of a history of a community under attack through slavery, apartheid, and the continued racial-ethnic and social-class oppression of contemporary South Africa. We quoted Angela

Gillian (1991) in chapter 1 explaining that according to postcolonial feminists, "the separation of sexism from the political, economic, and racial is a strategy of elites. As such, it becomes a tool to confuse the real issues around which most of the world's women struggle" (p. 229). The women in our study remind us of the importance of taking Gillian's advice. Activists and policy makers will need to look at both gender injustice and all other oppressions to sort through the best way to move ahead. We cannot ignore the cruel treatment of women by the men closest to them. But in order to address that problem, we will need to pay attention to the ties of nation, race ethnicity, and social class that bind women to their partners.

Discourses of Women's Bodies

Another topic the women in our study tied to the issues of HIV is the problem of bodies. The women spoke about the appearance of their bodies, including how their bodies have changed shape or have become thinner and how they believe their beauty has faded. There seems to be no space for women living with HIV in a world permeated by rigid, exploitative, and oppressive beauty and body standards. The even larger problem remains that the women must exert precious resources and energy on the issue of the appearance of their bodies in order to maintain relationships with men and to avoid being further marginalized.

Women in general must often visibly display their femininity (which is embodied in the set of ideals set forth by the dominant culture) in order to compensate for any of their "unfeminine" characteristics (Rodin, 1993). This includes bodies affected by poverty and HIV. Forcing women to be preoccupied with their appearance is an effective way of oppressing women and maintaining a system of gender dominance (Kirk & Okazawa-Rey, 2004). In this study we find that it endangers women who are HIV positive and may need body-shape-changing ARVs but who also feel they must adhere to impossible beauty standards that are even more unattainable for them than they are for other women. If they choose ARVs, their bodies will be distorted from an "ideal" womanly shape. If they do not choose ARVs, their emaciated bodies will also be "unwomanly." Either way they will feel as if they are not quite women and will fret about how others see them and the changes in their bodies. Their fretting is emotionally distressing and creates physical stress as well, which hinders their ability to stay as healthy as possible.

On a more hopeful note, Reischer and Koo (2004) remind us that because the bodies of women are the site of oppression, they may also be the site of empowerment. Persson (2005) describes an example of this in the resistance against stigma and exclusion brought on by the visible side effects of ARVs in communities of gay men in Australia. The men in the Persson study exhibit "a kind of defiant 'normalization' of HIV" (p. 250) when they create a sense of "brotherhood" by being comfortable and open about their own body-shape changes. Although the resistance exemplified in the Persson study has been achieved by men, it shows that the body can be a site of successful resistance against systems of gender.

Our study reveals that women, too, can challenge gender norms by experiencing their bodies as a site of resistance. Women like Elaine, for example, are actively resisting the necessity to adhere to a certain set of standards that excludes and shames the bodies of women living with HIV. Toward the end of our interview, Elaine explained how she is becoming prouder to be an HIV-positive activist and is feeling better in her own thin but powerful body. December 1 is World AIDS Day, and Elaine has a T-shirt she wears commemorating this day. The shirt says "HIV positive" on the front, playing on the double meaning of the word "positive" in the slogan.

> Like the lady who said to me when I got that blue sweater [T-shirt] on at that December the 1st—last year, "Oh, this is a shit sweater! Why did you have to put on that sweater?" I said to her, "You know what? You don't know what you're talking, because why? This sweater I represent all the people living with HIV." I said to her, "You don't know. I represent the people living with HIV and those who have passed away with HIV." I said, "That's why I'm wearing this today and it makes me look beautiful. Why did you come and tell me this is stupid nonsense shit? It's not that. You don't know what you talking about!" No, I know how to . . . I don't know if because I went to the support group or I learned about HIV. Now I'm like nobody's gonna tell me—I've got an answer for everybody.

Real Women/Real Humans

Through discourses of work and relationships with men, the imperative of disclosure, doing care work for children and for men who may be abusive, and body considerations, the women we interviewed drew upon an overarching discourse of femininity. Their words are about what they believe or what they have heard real women must do and feel and look like in order to be "normal women." Their words told us of the dehumanizing character of the dominant discourse of HIV. But they also told us of how these marginalized women grapple with various issues and assert themselves as truly women and truly human.

The women emphasized their need to work, not only as an act of providing for their families and having a sense of purpose in their lives but also because it is a normative and highly regarded behavior for Coloured women in South Africa. The discourse of disclosure can also be seen as a pressure for women to normalize in the sense that it is drawn upon by the medical and HIV activist communities in South Africa as a necessity for people living with HIV. As well, the women underscored the necessity of doing care work for children and men, even though they may be abusive. Care work is a type of work that a patriarchal system pressures or forces women to perform, and it is considered a feminine duty, but it is also a way of remaining connected, useful members of their households and communities. It is a reflection of a world where gender injustice is not the only problem, and it is not something that can be addressed in isolation from communities and couples bound together by race ethnicity and social class. Caring for and loving men further normalizes women, because it "fits" within the ideals of emotional relationships. Feeling and expressing love, in spite of everything else—the work, the abuse, the betrayal—creates an appearance and perhaps a real experience of love, which is identified with being human and being part of the human community. Finally, the discourse of the appearance of their body in all of its changes that may or may not be due to HIV and ARVs emerged as a great concern. Adhering to feminine beauty and body ideals is a way for marginalized women to appear as healthy and normal. The women voiced their struggle to conform to Northern expectations of beauty as well as Southern ideals of a healthy body as being big. They mourned the loss of their beauty. They also described their frustration, however, with others who criticize them when they don't meet the goal of being beautiful.

Emphasized femininity and normalizing discourses emerged as tools by which women attempt to bring themselves back from the edge of poverty and HIV. At times these methods are problematic because they are the very tools with which the systems that oppress women maintain the status quo. Nevertheless, they also are sites of resistance, enabling women to use standards of femininity to their advantage and pull themselves back into the normal world.

Global Lessons from Local Voices

These discourses around work and men, disclosure, care work, and body image reflect the concerns women have with being pushed to the very edge of society because of racism, violence against women, poverty, and HIV. This marginalization means women must draw themselves back into the realm of acceptance and normalcy for their own survival and well-being. This "coming back to normal" requires women to emphasize certain feminine behaviors that tell society they are not "HIV," but, rather, they are normal women. These ideas, although they are in some ways related to issues in the literature on gender and HIV, have not been widely recognized or researched.

The predominant scientific and academic discourses on gender and HIV emerge from the Global North. Those discourses have significant effects on how the virus and those living with it are treated globally. The literature tells a story from the point of view of scholars and policy makers, mostly based in the Global North, about what should be done about the "HIV problem." Northern scholars have dominated the protocols for both the development of tools used to prevent HIV infection as well as the ideas and practices that deal with the people who have already been infected (as well, they have monopolized the resources with which to implement these protocols). There is an overarching belief reflected in scholarly work that knowledge is the central, almost single factor in "combating HIV." For example, in HIV support groups all over the world, including South Africa, it is common procedure to hold workshops for members about using condoms, healthy cooking, and personal hygiene. But these programs have fallen far short of effectively addressing the issues.

The statistics show that HIV prevalence and infection rates in most parts of the world are not decreasing or even slowing down significantly; in fact, they are rising for women. A shift in our thinking is essential to figure out this problem. We must determine the political and social barriers that prevent us from supporting people who are HIV positive and from stopping the spread of the virus. In order to do that we must listen to those who are most closely affected. We must replace the voices of the power structures with the voices of people who have been invisible or marginalized (Fraser, 1996). In the world of academia, we have established a huge body of literature from "above," and now, because of the continuing escalation of HIV, it appears that finally we will be forced to try a new approach, which is the approach from "below" (Mies, 1983, p. 120).

In the debates such as the one over the ABCs and GEM (see chapter 1), the international community of scholars and policy makers have recognized that gender plays a role in women's experiences regarding their risk of becoming infected and the subsequent specific difficulties they may face in dealing with HIV infection. The discourses from the voices from below in our study reveal that gender emerges in a range of additional ways as a critical issue. The women in our study seem to perceive their contracting and living with HIV as amounting to a departure from the hegemonic norms of femininity. As a result, they draw on discourses of emphasized femininity as a way to compensate for their lack of conformity to particular gendered expectations. These discoveries are new and have not been attended to as yet by either scholars or policy makers.

Goffman (1988, p. 6) asserts that through "gender displays" we convey our gender to others in a way that makes our gendered behaviors appear to be natural. Connell (1987) uses the term "emphasized femininity" to describe femininity that dominates our thoughts, behaviors, and expectations for what real women are. She writes, "One form [of femininity] is defined around compliance with this subordination and is oriented to accommodating the interests and desires of men. I call this 'emphasized femininity'" (p. 183). Emphasized femininity in many places, including South Africa, is characterized by displays of nurturance and selflessness. The women we interviewed exaggerated their femininity in specific ways in their frequent talk of what they consider feminine behaviors and expectations, such as working, being in monogamous relationships with men, doing care work, and worrying about their appearance.

The way the women in our study have dealt with certain aspects of HIV, however, is ironic. They are forced to rely on the exaggeration of specific feminine gender expectations to bring themselves to "normal." Emphasized femininity is a dangerous tool in this case, as it locks women into roles and behaviors that are ultimately detrimental because they disempower women by forcing them to spend energy trying to reach goals of "normalcy." For example, the women we interviewed shoulder the burden of the care and responsibility in their community in dealing with HIV and other issues, because sexist ideals expect women to do this kind of work. Emphasized femininity in this case is not in the best interest of women whose own health needs are ignored or threatened because of the care work burden. In addition, striving toward those goals means they endanger their health, subject themselves to enormous stress, and even chain themselves to remaining in violent relationships.

All expressions of femininity, however, are not the same (Connell, 1987). Some expressions of femininity "are defined by strategies of resistance or forms of non-compliance. Others, again, are defined by complex strategic combinations of compliance, resistance, and co-operation" (pp. 183–184). In our study women also fall into these other categories. They are challenging power structures and dominant discourses by calling less for workshops on how to use condoms and dress bed-sores and more for change at the community level. Most significantly, they are calling for a community that is supportive of human rights and women regardless of their HIV status. Furthermore, they described a community that recognizes women living with HIV as normal people—real humans and real women—who are trying to live life and happen to be living with a common disease. This is not to say that the women we interviewed have perfect lives except for the fact that they are living with HIV. In fact, all of the women interviewed have very difficult lives as they struggle to support themselves and their children and partners with few resources and little to no money. These difficulties highlight broader issues of poverty and marginalization affecting the lives of women living with the virus (Fraser, 1997).

Striving to be real "normal" women is contradictory. It includes oppression, but it also includes opportunities and acts of resistance. Our goal must be to tease out these strategies of resistance and find ways to enhance and support them. In order to do so, we will need to understand the links between gender and HIV.

Gender Mainstreaming in HIV

Researchers and activists alike could ask, "What about HIV does not relate to women, and what social sectors are not affected by HIV?" and "What aspects of HIV are not shaped by gender?" In speaking about their lives, the women in our study pointed to the organization of gender in several social milieus—paid work, marriage, love, care work, and ideals of beauty—as being critical to their experience with HIV. Despite the facts that poor people and women are increasingly vulnerable to HIV, that the virus has spread into all social sectors and the infrastructures of many countries, and that gender and HIV are strongly connected, HIV is still predominantly viewed as a biomedical problem (Elsey, Tolhurst & Theobald, 2005). The issues of gender and HIV are often still viewed as areas of concern separate from each other as well as detached from other social issues (Tiessen, 2005). One possible way to tie the issues together in our thinking and in our policy making is gender mainstreaming. The idea of gender mainstreaming as a way to address many social issues came to light in 1995 with the adoption of the Beijing Platform for Action at the UN International Conference on Women. According to Elsey and her colleagues (2005), gender mainstreaming "aims to ensure that women's, as well as men's concerns and priorities influence the 'mainstream' activities of development, including resource allocation, policy and legislation formulation, and program or project planning, implementation, monitoring and evaluation" (p. 991). When HIV is added to the equation, it means the effects of the virus must be taken into consideration in these same ways.

Gender mainstreaming in HIV is just beginning to emerge as a strategy to uphold human rights that could be more successful than the current strategies to eliminate the spread of the virus and support those people living with HIV. Gender mainstreaming efforts have begun, for example, in sub-Saharan Africa. These efforts, however, have not been without problems. Unfortunately, gender mainstreaming regarding HIV has been misinterpreted by governments and policy makers who believe that by adding more women to the predetermined structures in government, business, and other social sectors, gender mainstreaming, and subsequently HIV mainstreaming, has taken place (Tiessen, 2005; True, 2003). Increasing the numbers of women receiving social support and ARVs is a positive step; however, it does not address or get at the root of the problem of HIV. Gender mainstreaming in HIV is much more than adding women and stirring; it also must aim to fundamentally change the way that governments and social sectors are structured. It must seek to "reinvent processes of policy formulation and implementation across all issue areas at all levels from a gender-differentiated perspective" (True, 2003, p. 369). If HIV is to be eliminated and treated successfully, it is essential that HIV be recognized as a social problem and that the gender norms that currently put women at disadvantaged positions be overturned.

Gender mainstreaming in HIV might be a productive way forward, but before it can be effective it has to take into consideration exactly what changes need to take place. Unfortunately, the largest proportion of the body of literature on HIV is not focused on the virus as a social problem. Many studies involve more men than women and then generalize their conclusions. Alternatively, "women's issues" are addressed in a way that further stigmatizes women living with the virus. There are few studies that allow women living with HIV to voice their concerns about the virus and about their lives holistically. There is also the problem of HIV research painting women as victims (Oinas & Jungar, 2005) and not adequately highlighting the ways women are able to resist this victim status and offer themselves and other women positions of power. Increasingly, however, more women activists living with HIV, like the women in the International Community of Women Living with HIV/AIDS (ICW), are speaking up about the concerns and experiences of HIV-positive women (Bell, 2005). The women in the ICW point out that laws, programs, and policies are "often determined by people who do not understand the realities in which HIV-positive women live their lives" (p. 71). In addition, Seidel (1993) argues that the activist discourse is one in which the voices of African researchers and professionals need to be heard in the international HIV arena. Bell (2005) goes further and calls for the need to hear the voices of women in determining the "direction of policies and programs" (p. 71).

This book has presented empirical evidence to convey the priorities and concerns in the words of women living with HIV in contribution to the needed body of literature surrounding this virus as a gendered social problem. This research, and further research along the same lines, must be utilized in the creation and restructuring of policy and programs for both women and men living with HIV. Most important, the process, as well as the findings, of this study and studies like it are ways for women who have been marginalized to be empowered and to demand their voices be heard.

Key Lessons: Bringing the Margins to the Center

The most important lesson learned from our study is that women on the margins have something different to say about HIV. Their stories reveal issues that are not widely discussed among policy makers and scholars. Their insights reveal that HIV is truly a complex issue that touches on myriad issues for those who are infected and affected by the virus, and their ideas point to the precise factors in that complexity. Their insights also reveal some of the specific ways that gender is tightly linked to all of these factors.

In particular, in the case of low-income Coloured women in South Africa, we have learned that government policy on health care and welfare, intimate heterosexual relationships, care work, notions of love, interpersonal violence, the power of racial-ethnic and social-class ties in couples, family relationships between mothers and children, poverty, ARVs, and support groups are all essential pieces of the picture that must be taken into account if we are to really tackle the problem of HIV.

References

Adam, B., & Sears, A. (1996). *Experiencing HIV: Personal, family and work relationships.* New York, NY: Columbia University Press.

Adamsen, L. (2002). From victim to agent: The clinical and social significance of self-help group participation for people with life-threatening diseases. *Scandinavian Journal of Caring Sciences,* 16(3), 224–231.

Adhikari, M. (2006). Hope, fear, shame, frustration: Continuity and change in the expression of coloured identity in white supremacist South Africa, 1910–1994. *Journal of Southern African Studies,* 32(3), 467–487.

———. (2011). *The anatomy of a South African genocide: The extermination of the Cape San people.* Athens, OH: Ohio University Press.

Ashton, E., Vosvick, M., Chesney, M., Gore-Felton, C., Koopman, C., O'Shea, K., Maldonado, J., Bachmann, M., Israelski, D., Flamm, J., & Spiegel, G. (2005). Social support and maladaptive coping as predictors of change in physical health symptoms among persons living with HIV/AIDS. *AIDS Patient Care and STDs,* 19(9), 587–598.

Austin, S. B. (1989). AIDS and Africa: United States media and racist fantasy. *Cultural Critique,* 14, 129–152.

Avert. (2005). *President's Emergency Plan for AIDS Relief (PEPFAR).* Retrieved from http://www.avert.org/pepfar.htm.

———. (2010a). *The origin of HIV and AIDS and the first cases of AIDS.* Retrieved from http://www.avert.org/origin-aids-hiv.htm.

———. (2010b). *Reducing the price of HIV/AIDS treatments.* Retrieved from http://www.avert.org/generic.htm.

———. (2010c). *HIV and AIDS home-based care.* Retrieved from http://www.avert.org/aids-home-care.htm.

———. (2012). *HIV and AIDS in South Africa.* Retrieved from http://www.avert.org/aidssouthafrica.htm.

Bakken, S., Holzemer, W. L., Brown, M. A., Powell-Cope, G. M., Turner, J. G., Inouye, J., Nokes, K. M., & Corless, I. B. (2000). Relationships between perception of engagement with health care provider and demographic characteristics, health status, and adherence to therapeutic regimens in persons with HIV/AIDS. *AIDS Patient Care and STDS,* 14(4), 189–197.

Barker, G., Ricardo, C., & Nascimento, M. (2007). *Engaging men and boys in changing gender-based inequity in health: Evidence from programme interventions.* World Health Organization: Geneva.

BBC. (1980). *Panorama: Walking on coals: The white tribe of Africa.* Retrieved from http://www.bbc.co.uk/archive/apartheid/7212.shtml.

———. (2000). *Mandela's AIDS speech: Excerpts.* Retrieved from http://news.bbc.co.uk/2/hi/world/monitoring/media_reports/833996.stm.

———. (2010). *Anti-retrovirals could halt Aids spread in five years.* Retrieved from http://news.bbc.co.uk/go/pr/fr/-/2/hi/science/nature/8526690.stm.

Beck, R. B. (2000). *The history of South Africa.* London, England: Greenwood Press.

Beckett, A., & Rutan, J. S. (1990). Treating persons with ARC and AIDS in group psychotherapy. *International Journal of Group Psychotherapy, 40*(1), 19–29.

Bell, E. (2005). Advocacy training by the international community of women living with HIV/AIDS. *Gender and Development, 13*(3), 70–79.

Benton, S. (2007). Government provision of ARVs nearly doubles in nine months. *BUA News.* Retrieved from http://www.buanews.gov.za/news/07/07050815451012.

Beyers, C. (2008). The cultural politics of "community" and citizenship in the District Six Museum, Cape Town. *Anthropologica 50*(2), 359–373.

Biehl, J. G. (2007). *Will to live: AIDS therapies and the politics of survival.* Princeton, NJ: Princeton University Press.

Bloomberg Brief. (2012). *South African unemployment rate quarterly.* Retrieved from http://www.bloomberg.com/quote/SAUERATQ:IND.

Blumenreich, M. (2003). Confidentiality, equity and silence: A critical look at school policy and HIV positive children. *Equity and Excellence in Education, 36*(1), 64–70.

Boonzaier, F. (2001). *Woman abuse: Exploring women's narratives of violence and resistance in Mitchell's Plain.* Master's thesis. University of Cape Town, Cape Town, South Africa.

———. (2005). Women abuse in South Africa: A brief contextual analysis. *Feminism & Psychology, 15*(1), 99–103.

Boonzaier, F., & de la Rey, C. (2004). Woman abuse: The construction of gender in women and men's narratives of violence. *South African Journal of Psychology, 34*(3), 443–463.

Boonzaier, F., & Shefer, T. (2006). Gendered research. In T. Shefer, F. Boonzaier & P. Kiguwa (Eds.), *The gender of psychology* (pp. 3–11), Cape Town, South Africa: University of Cape Town Press.

Booth, K. M. (2004). *Local women, global science: Fighting AIDS in Kenya.* Bloomington, IN: University of Indiana Press.

Bordo, S. (1993). *Unbearable weight: Feminism, western culture, and the body.* Berkeley, CA: University of California Press.

Botshabelo, M., & Nakanyane, S. (2006). *Women in the South African labour market.* Department of Labour, Republic of South Africa. Retrieved from https://www.labour.gov.za/downloads/documents/useful-documents/labour-market-research-and-statistics/Labour%20Market%20Research%20-%20Women%20in%20the%20South%20African%20Labour%20Market%201995%20-%202005.pdf.

Brashers, D. E., Haas, S. M., Klingle, R. S., & Neidig, J. L. (2000). Collective AIDS activism and individual's perceived self-advocacy in physician-patient communication. *Human Communication Research, 26*(3), 372–402.

Brief, D. J., Bollinger, A. R., Vielhauer, M. J., Berger-Greenstein, J. A., Morgan, E. E., Brady, S. M., Buondonno, L. M., & Keane, T. M. (2004). Understanding the interface of HIV, trauma, post-traumatic stress disorder, and substance use and its implications for health outcomes. *AIDS Care, 16*(Supplement 1), 97–121.

Brown, K. S., Marean, C. W., Herries, A. I. R., Jacobs, Z., Tribolo, C., Braun, D., Roberts, D. L., Meyer, M. C., & Bernatchez, J. (2009). Fire as an engineering tool of early modern humans. *Science, 325*(5942), 859–862.

Budlender, D. J. (2004). *Why should we care about unpaid care work?* Harare, Zimbabwe: United Nations Development Fund.

Butler, J. (2006). *Gender trouble: Feminism and the subversion of identity.* New York, NY: Routledge.

Castle, S. (2004). Rural children's attitudes to people with HIV/AIDS in Mali: The causes of stigma. *Culture, Health & Sexuality,* 6, 1–18.

Catz, S. L., Heckman, T. G., Kochman, A., & DiMarco, M. (2001). Rates and correlates of HIV treatment adherence among late middle-aged and older adults living with HIV disease. *Psychology of Health and Medicine,* 6, 47–58.

Chacham, A. S., Maia, M. B., Greco, M., Silva, A. P., & Greco, D. B. (2007). Autonomy and susceptibility to HIV/AIDS among young women living in a slum in Belo Horizonte, Brazil. *AIDS Care,* 19, S12–S22.

Chesney, M. A. (2003). Adherence to HAART regimens. *AIDS Patient Care and STDS,* 17, 169–177.

Children's Act No. 38 of 2005. (2005). Republic of South Africa. Retrieved from http://ci.org.za/depts/ci/pubs/rights/bills/Children%27sAct38of2005.pdf.

Chireshe, E., & Chireshe, R. (2011). Monogamous marriage in Zimbabwe: An insurance against HIV and AIDS? *Agenda,* 87, 93–101.

Chirimuuta, R., & Chirimuuta, R. (1989). *AIDS, Africa and racism.* London, England: Free Association Books.

Choice on Termination of Pregnancy Act. (1996). Retrieved from http://www.info.gov.za/acts/1996/a92-96.pdf.

Chung, J. Y., & Magraw, M. M. (1992). A group approach to psychosocial issues faced by HIV-positive women. *Hospital and Community Psychiatry,* 43(9), 891–894.

Cohen, Robin. (2007). Creolization and cultural globalization: The soft sounds of fugitive power. *Globalizations* 4(3), 369–384.

Cole, J., & Thomas, L. (2009). *Love in Africa.* Chicago, IL: University of Chicago Press.

Collins, E. J., Burgoyne, R. W., Wagner, C. A., Abbey, S. E., Halman, M. H., Nur, M. L., & Walmsley, S. L. (2006). Lipodystrophy severity does not contribute to HAART nonadherence. *AIDS and Behavior,* 10, 273–277.

Collins, P. H. (2000). *Black feminist thought: Knowledge, consciousness and the politics of empowerment.* New York, NY: Routledge.

———. (2004). *Black sexual politics: African Americans, gender and the new racism.* New York, NY: Routledge.

Connell, R. W. (1987). *Gender and power: Society, the person and sexual politics.* Cambridge, UK: Polity Press.

Cooper, D., Harries, J., Myer, L., Orner, P., Bracken, H., & Zweigenthal, V. (2007). "Life is still going on": Reproductive intentions among HIV positive women and men in South Africa. *Social Science & Medicine,* 65(10), 274–283.

Corey, G. (2000). *Theory and practice of group counseling,* (5th ed.). Belmont, CA. Wadsworth/Thomson Learning.

Csaky, C. (2008). *No one to turn to: The under reporting of child sexual abuse and exploitation by aid workers and peacekeepers.* London, England: Save the Children. Retrieved from http://www.un.org/en/pseataskforce/docs/no_one_to_turn_under_reporting_of_child_sea_by_aid_workers.pdf.

Deacon, H., Stephney, I., & Prosalendis, S. (2005). *Understanding HIV/AIDS stigma: A*

146 | *References*

theoretical and methodological analysis. Cape Town, South Africa: Human Sciences Research Council Research Monograph.

Delahanty, D. L., Bogart, L. M., & Figler, J. L. (2004). Post-traumatic stress disorder symptoms, salivary cortisol, medication adherence, and CD4 levels in HIV-positive individuals. *AIDS Care, 16,* 247–261.

Department of Labour Employment Equity Act, Act No.55, Republic of South Africa. (1998). Code of good practice on key aspects of HIV/AIDS and employment. Retrieved from http://www.exclaim.co.za/fileadmin/September_2011/Document%203.pdf.

Department of Social Development, Republic of South Africa. (2006). *Report on incentive structures of social assistance grants in South Africa.* Retrieved from http://www.socdev.gov.za/documents/2006/incent.doc.

Derlega, V. J., Winstead, B. A., Greene, K., Serovich, J., & Elwood, W. N. (2002). Perceived HIV-related stigma and HIV disclosure to relationship partners after finding out about the seropositive diagnosis. *Journal of Health Psychology, 7,* 415–432.

DeVault, M. L.. (1999). *Liberating method: Feminism and social research.* Philadelphia, PA: Temple University Press.

Dobash, R. E., & Dobash, R. P. (1979). *Violence against wives. A case against patriarchy.* New York, NY: Free Press.

Dooling, W. (2007). *Slavery, emancipation and colonial rule in South Africa.* Athens, OH: Ohio University Press.

Doyal, L., & Anderson, J. (2006). HIV-positive African women surviving in London: Report of a qualitative study. *Gender & Development, 14,* 95–104.

Dunkle, K. L., Jewkes, R. K., Brown, H. C., Gray, G. E., McIntyre, J. A., & Harlow, S. D. (2004). Transactional sex among women in Soweto, South Africa: Prevalence, risk factors and association with HIV infection. *Social Science & Medicine, 59,* 1581–1592.

Dworkin, S., & Erhardt, A. (2007). Going beyond "ABC" to include "GEM": Critical reflections on progress in the HIV/AIDS epidemic. *American Journal of Public Health, 97*(1), 13–18.

Eisenstein, H. (2009). *Feminism seduced: How global elites use women's labor and ideas to exploit the world.* London, England: Paradigm Press.

Ellece, S. E. (2011). "Be a fool like me": Gender construction in the marriage advice ceremony in Botswana—A critical discourse analysis. *Agenda, 87,* 43–52.

Elsey, H., Tolhurst, R., & Theobald, S. (2005). Mainstreaming HIV/AIDS in development sectors: Have we learnt the lessons from gender mainstreaming? *AIDS Care, 17,* 988–998.

Elson, D. (2005). *Unpaid work, the millennium development goals, and capital accumulation.* Proceedings from Conference on Unpaid Work and the Economy: Gender, Poverty, and the Millennium Development Goals.

Faludi, S. (2006). *Backlash: The undeclared war against American women.* New York, NY: Three Rivers Press.

Farmer, P. (1992). *AIDS and accusations: Haiti and the geography of blame.* Berkeley, CA: University of California Press.

Fataar, A. (2007). Identity formation and communal negotiations in a "bounded" geographic space: The formative discourses of Muslim teachers in apartheid Cape Town. *Journal of Muslim Minority Affairs 27*(1), 155–170.

Fausto-Sterling, A. (2012). Bodies with histories: The new search for the biology of race. *Boston Review*. Retrieved from http://www.bostonreview.net/BR37.3/anne_fausto -sterling_biology_race.php.

Fife, B. L., & Wright, E. R. (2000). The dimensionality of stigma: A comparison of its impact on the self of persons with HIV/AIDS and cancer. *Journal of Health and Social Behavior*, 41, 50–67.

Fisher, B., & Tronto, J. (1990). Towards a feminist theory of caring. In E. K. Abel and M. K. Nelson (Eds.), *Circles of care: Work and identity in women's lives* (pp. 35–61). Albany, NY: State University of New York Press.

Fleischman, J. (2006). *Integrating reproductive health and HIV/AIDS programs— Strategic opportunities for PEPFAR*. Washington, DC: Center for Strategic and International Studies.

Flick, U. (2006). *An introduction to qualitative research* (3rd ed.). London, England: Sage.

Folkman, S., Chesney, M., & Christopher-Richards, A. (1994). Stress and coping in care-giving partners of men with AIDS. *Psychiatric Clinic of North America*, 1, 35–53.

Foster, S. B., Stevens, P., & Hall, J. (1994). Offering support groups services for lesbians living with HIV. *Women and Therapy*, 15, 69–83.

Foucault, M. (1978). *The history of sexuality: An introduction* (Vol. 1). New York, NY: Vintage.

———. (1980). *Power/knowledge: Selected interviews and other writings, 1972–1977*. New York, NY: Pantheon.

Fraser, Nancy. (1997). *Justice interruptus: Critical reflections on the "post-socialist condi-tion"* Philadelphia, PA: Routledge.

Friedland, J., Renwick, R., & McColl, M. (1996). Coping and social support as determi-nants of quality of life in HIV/AIDS. *AIDS Care*, 8, 15–31.

Frye, M. (1990). A response to "lesbian ethics." *Hypatia*, 5(3), 132–137.

———. (2010). *Oppression*. Retrieved from http://feminsttheoryreadinggroup.wordpress .com/2010/11/23/marilyn-frye-the-politics-of-reality-oppression.

Gallo, R. C. (2006). A reflection of HIV/AIDS research after 25 years. *Retrovirology*, 3, 1–7.

Gavey, N. (1989). Feminist poststructuralism and discourse analysis: Contributions to feminist psychology. *Psychology of Women Quarterly*, 13, 459–475.

Gillett, H. J., & Parr, J. (2010). Disclosure among HIV-positive women: The role of HIV/ AIDS support groups in rural Kenya. *African Journal of AIDS Research*, 9(4), 337–344.

Gillian, A. (1991). Women's equality and national liberation. In C. Mohanty, A. Russo, & L. Torres (Eds.), *Third world women and the politics of feminism* (pp. 215–236). Bloomington, IN: Indiana University Press.

Gillies, J. (2004). Reframing the HIV debate in developing countries IV: Does ethics have anything to offer? *Rural and Remote Health*. Retrieved from www.rrh.org.au.

Goffman, E. (1963). *Stigma: Notes on the management of a spoiled identity*. Englewood Cliffs, NJ: Prentice Hall.

———. (1988). *Gender advertisements* (Rev. ed.). New York, NY: Harper.

Gonzalez J. S., Batchelder, A. W., Psaros, C., Safren, S. A. (2011). Depression and HIV/ AIDS treatment nonadherence: A review and meta-analysis. *Journal of Acquired Immune Deficiency Syndrome*, 58, 181–187.

Govender, P. (2009). SA won't meet ARV roll-out target, says Motsoaledi. *Mail & Guard-*

ian online 12 (September 15): 11. Retrieved from http://www.mg.co.za/article /2009–09–15-sa-wont-meet-arv-rollout-target-says-motsoaledi.

Green, G. (1993). Editorial review: Support and HIV. *AIDS Care,* 5, 87–103.

Grunebaum, H., & Robins, S. (2001). Crossing the colour line: Mediating the ambiguities of belonging and identity. In Z. Erasmus (Ed.), *Coloured by history, shaped by place: New perspectives on Coloured identities in Cape Town* (pp. 159–172). Cape Town, South Africa: Kwela Books.

Guedes, A. (2004). *Addressing gender-based violence from the reproductive health/HIV sector, a literature review and analysis.* United States Agency for International Development (USAID).

Gunsaullus, J. A. (2006). *The "Condom Lady" speaks: Female sexuality discourses and HIV prevention in community-based organisations* (Doctoral dissertation, State University of New York at Albany, 2006). Dissertation Abstracts International, 67/01, 350.

Hader, S. L., Smith, D. K., Moore, J. S., & Holmberg, S. D. (2001). HIV infection in women in the United States: Status at the millennium. *Journal of the American Medical Association,* 285, 1186–1192.

Hallman, K. (2005). Gendered socioeconomic conditions and HIV risk behaviours among young people in South Africa. *African Journal of AIDS Research,* 4, 37–50.

Hardy, C., & Richter, M. (2006). Disability grants or antiretrovirals? A quandary for people with HIV/AIDS in South Africa. *African Journal of AIDS Research,* 5, 85–96.

Harrington, S. (1997). Women and AIDS: Bodily representations, political repercussions. In D. S. Wilson & C. M. Laennec (Eds.), *Bodily discursions, genders, representations, technologies* (pp. 201–219). Albany, NY: State University of New York Press.

Harrington Meyer, M., Herd, P., & Michel, S. (2000). Introduction. In M. Harrington Meyer (Ed.), *Care work: Gender, labor, and the welfare state* (p. 104). New York, NY: Routledge.

Hays, R. B., Chauncey, S., & Tobey, L. A. (1990). The social support networks of gay men with AIDS. *Journal of Community Psychology,* 18, 374–18,385.

Hedge, B., & Glover, L. F. (1990). Group intervention with HIV seropositive patients and their partners. *AIDS Care,* 2 (2), 147–154.

Hendricks, C. (2001). Ominous liaisons: Tracing the interface between "race" and sex at the Cape. In Z. Erasmus (Ed.), *Coloured by history, shaped by place.* Cape Town, South Africa: Kwela Books.

Hirsch, J., Wardlow, H., Smith, D., Phinney, H. M., Parikh, S., & Nathanson, C. A. (2009). *The secret: Love, marriage, and HIV.* Nashville, TN: Vanderbilt University Press.

Hollway, W. (1983). Heterosexual sex: Power and desire for the other. In S. Cartledge & J. Ryan (Eds.), *Sex and love: New thoughts on old contradictions* (pp. 124–140). London, England: Women's Press.

Hoosen, S., & Collins, A. (2004). Sex, sexuality and sickness: Discourses of gender and HIV/AIDS among KwaZulu-Natal women. *South African Journal of Psychology,* 34, 487–505.

Huff, J. L. (2001). A "horror of corpulence": Interrogating Bantingism and mid-nineteenth-century fat phobia. In J. E. Braziel & K. LeBesco (Eds.), *Bodies out of* bounds: *Fatness and transgression* (pp. 39–59). Berkeley, CA: University of California Press.

Hunter, M. (2010). *Love in the time of AIDS.* Bloomington, IN: Indiana University Press.

Hurley, E., Coutsoudis, A., Giddy, J., Knight, S. E., Loots, E., & Esterhuizen, T. M. (2011). Weight evolution and perceptions of adults living with HIV following initiation of antiretroviral therapy in a South African urban setting. *South African Medical Journal,* 101(9), 645–650.

Issiaka, S., Cartoux, M., Ky-Zerbo, O., Tiendrebeogo, S., Meda, N., Dabis, F., & Van de Perre, P. (2001). Living with HIV: Women's experience in Burkina Faso, West Africa. *AIDS Care,* 13, 20–29.

Jeppe, S. (2001). Coloured, Malay, Muslim. In Z. Erasmus (Ed.) *Coloured by history, shaped by place.* Cape Town, South Africa: Kwela Books.

Jones, L. (2005). Childcare in poor urban settlements in Swaziland in an era of HIV/AIDS. *African Journal of AIDS Research,* 4(3), 161–171.

Kalichman, S. C., Sikkema, K. J., & Somlai, A. (1996). People living with HIV infection who attend and do not attend support groups: A pilot study of needs, characteristics and experiences. *AIDS Care,* 8(5), 589–599.

Kalichman, S. C., & Simbayi, L. C. (2004). Traditional beliefs about the cause of AIDS and AIDS-related stigma in South Africa. *AIDS Care,* 16, 572–581.

kaNdlondlo, M. (2011). When sacrificing self is the only way out: A tribute to my mother. *Agenda,* 87, 15–21.

Kelly, K., & Mzizi, T. (2005). The implications of ART for local AIDS care and support programs. *AIDS Bulletin,* 14, 1–8.

Kim, J. C. (2002). *Rape and HIV post-exposure prophylaxis (PEP).* Paper presented to the South African Gender-Based Violence and Health Conference, April 17–19.

Kimberly, J. A., Serovich, J. M., & Greene, K. (1995). Disclosure of HIV positive status: Five women's stories. *Family Relations,* 44, 316–322.

Kirk, G., & Okazawa-Rey, M. (2004). *Women's lives: Multicultural perspectives.* New York, NY: McGraw Hill.

Kishor, S. (2005). *Violence against women: A statistical overview, challenges and gaps in data collection and methodology and approaches for overcoming them.* UN Division for the Advancement of Women in collaboration with: Economic Commission for Europe (ECE) and World Health Organization (WHO) 14 April, 2005 Geneva Switzerland. Retrieved from http://www.un.org/womenwatch/daw/egm /vaw-stat-2005/docs/expert-papers/Kishor.pdf.

Kistner, U. (2003).*Gender based violence and HIV in South Africa: A literature review. South Africa.* Centre for AIDS Development and Research and Evaluation (CADRE)/Department of Health.

Klitzman, R. L., Kirshenbaum, S. B., Dodge, B., Remien, R. H., Ehrhardt, A. A., Johnson, M. O., Kittel, L. E., Daya, S., Morkin, S. F., Kelly, J., Lightfoot, M., Rotheram-Borus, M. J., & The NIMH Healthy Living Trial Group. (2004). Intricacies and inter-relationships between HIV disclosure and HAART: A qualitative study. *AIDS Care,* 16, 628–640.

Knox, M. D. (1998). HIV community mental health services. In M. D. Knox and C. H. Sparks (Eds.) *HIV and community mental healthcare* (pp. 118). Baltimore, MD: Johns Hopkins University Press.

Kole, S. (2008). *Disease as development: Globalization and the political economy of HIV/*

AIDS in India. Proceedings from the 49th Annual Meetings of ISA in San Francisco, CA, March 26.

Kron, J. (2012). In Uganda, an AIDS success story comes undone. *New York Times,* August 2, 2012. Retrieved from http://www.nytimes.com/2012/08/03/world/africa/in-uganda-an-aids-success-story-comes-undone.html.

Kurz, D. (2001). Violence against women by intimate partners. In D. Vannoy (Ed.), *Gender Mosaics* (pp. 205–215). Los Angeles, CA: Roxbury Publishing.

Lekas, H. M., Siegel, K., & Schrimshaw, E. W. (2006). Continuities and discontinuities in the experiences of felt and enacted stigma among women with HIV/AIDS. *Qualitative Health Research,* 16, 1165–1190.

Lewis, S. (2006, August). *Remarks by Steven Lewis, UN special envoy for HIV/AIDS in Africa to the closing session of the XVI International AIDS Conference, Toronto.* Message posted to University of the Western Cape Listserv, archived at www.allafrica.com.

Li, L., Wu, S., Wu, Z., Sun, S., Cui, H., & Jia, M. (2006). Understanding family support for people living with HIV/AIDS in Yunnan, China. *AIDS & Behavior,* 10, 509–517.

Liamputtong, P., Haritavorn, N., & Kiatying-Angsulee, N. (2009). HIV and AIDS stigma and AIDS support groups: Perspectives from women living with HIV and AIDS in central Thailand. *Social Science & Medicine,* 69(6), 862–868.

Lorber, J., & Moore, L. J. (2002). *Gender and the social construction of illness.* New York, NY: Alta Mira Press.

———. (2007). *Gendered bodies: Feminist perspectives.* Los Angeles, CA: Roxbury Publishing.

Mahajan, A. P., Sayles, J. N., Patel, V. A., Remien, R. H., Sawires, S. R., Ortiz, D. J., Szekeres, G., Coates, T. J. 2008. Stigma in the HIV/AIDS epidemic: a review of the literature and recommendations for the way forward. *AIDS,* 22(S2), S67–S69.

Mail, P. D., & Matheny, S. C. (1989). Social services for people with AIDS: Needs and approaches. *AIDS,* 3(1), 273–278.

Makina, A. (2009). Caring for people with HIV: State policies and their dependence on women's unpaid work. *Gender & Development,* 17(2), 309–319.

Mandela, N. (2000). *Closing speech to the 13th International AIDS Conference* in Durban, July 14, 2000. Retrieved from http://www.afrol.com/Categories/Health/health011_mandela_speech.htm.

Mann, D. (2012, March 20). The most common cosmetic surgery in 2011 was . . . *WebMDhealthNews.* Retrieved from http://www.medicinenet.com/script/main/art.asp?articlekey=156124.

Mantell, J. E., Dworkin, S. L., Exner, T. M., Hoffman, S., Smith, J. A., & Susser, I. (2006). The promises and limitations of female-initiated methods of HIV/STI protection. *Social Science & Medicine,* 63, 1998–2009.

Marais, J. S. (1939/1968). *The cape Coloured people, 1652–1937.* Johannesburg, South Africa: Witwatersrand University Press.

Marso, L. J. (2010). Whatever happened to feminist critiques of marriage? Marriage and bourgeois respectability. *Politics & Gender,* 6(1), 145–153.

Martin, D. J., Riopelle, D., Steckart, J., Geshke, N., & Lin, S. (2001). Support group participation, HIV viral load and sexual-risk behaviour. *American Journal of Health Behavior,* 25(6), 513–527.

Marx, K., & Engels, F. (1848/2007). *The Communist Manifesto*. Minneapolis, MN: Fili-quarian.

Mbali, M., (2005). The Treatment Action Campaign and the history of rights-based, patient-driven HIV/AIDS activism in South Africa. In P. Jones & K. Stoke (Eds.) *Democratizing development: The politics of socio-economic rights in South Africa* (pp. 213–236). Netherlands: Martinus Nijhoff Publishers.

Mies, M. (1983). Toward a methodology for feminist research. In G. Bowles & R. Klein (Eds.), *Theories of women's studies* (pp. 117–139). London, England: Routledge and Kegan Paul.

Miles, M. B., & Huberman, A. M. (1994). *Qualitative data analysis: An expanded sourcebook* (2nd ed.). Thousand Oaks, CA: Sage.

Mill, J. E., & Anarfi, J. K. (2002). HIV risk environment for Ghanaian women: Challenges to prevention. *Social Science & Medicine, 54*, 325–337.

Mintz, S., & Kellogg, S. (1988). *Domestic revolutions: A social history of American family life*. New York, NY: Free Press.

Mohanty, C. T. (2006). US empire and the project of women's studies: Stories of citizenship, complicity and dissent. *Gender, Place and Culture, 13*, 1, 7–20,

Msibi, T. (2011). They are worried about me: I am worried too. *Agenda, 87*, 22–28.

Mundell, J. P. (2006). *The impact of structured supported groups for pregnant women living with HIV*. Unpublished dissertation. University of Pretoria, South Africa.

Mundell, J. P., Maretha, J. V., Visser, J., Makin, J. D., Kershaw, T. S., Forsyth, B. W., Jeffery, B., & Sikkema, K. J. (2011). The impact of structured support groups for pregnant South African women recently diagnosed HIV positive. *Women & Health, 51*(6), 546–565.

Mushunje, M. T. (2006). Challenges and opportunities for promoting the girl child's rights in the face of HIV/AIDS. *Gender and Development, 14*, 115–125.

Naples, N. A. (1987). Women, welfare and the politics of need interpretation. *Hypatia, 2*(1), 103–121.

———. (2003). *Feminism and methodology: Ethnography, discourse analysis, and activist research*. New York, NY: Routledge.

Nguyen, V. K. (2005). Antiretroviral globalism, biopolitics, and therapeutic citizenship. In A. Ong & S. J. Collier (Eds.), *Global assemblages: Technology, politics, and ethics as anthropological problems* (pp. 124–144). London, England: Blackwell.

Nokes, K., Chew, L., & Altman, C. (2003). Using a telephone support group for HIV-positive persons aged 50+ to increase social support and health-related knowledge. *AIDS Patient Care and STD's, 17*(7), 345–351.

Novello, A. C. (1992). *Surgeon General's address to an American Medical Association press conference on violence*. New York, NY.

Nuñes, J. A., Raymond, S. J., Nicholas, P. K., Leuner, J. D., & Webster, A. (1995). Social support, quality of life, immune function, and health in persons living with HIV. *Journal of Holistic Nursing, 13*, 174–198.

Nyamukapa, C., Foster, G., & Gregson, S. (2003). Orphans' household circumstances and access to education in a maturing epidemic in eastern Zimbabwe. *Journal of Social Development in Africa, 18*, 7–32.

Nyblade, L. C. (2006). Measuring HIV stigma: Existing knowledge and gaps. *Psychology, Health & Medicine, 11*, 335–345.

Odgen, J., Esim, S., & Grown, C. (2004). *Expanding the care continuum for HIV/AIDS: Bringing carers into focus. Horizons Report.* Washington, DC: Population Council and International Center for Research on Women.

Office of the Law Revision Counsel. (2010). *"United States Code" United States Leadership against HIV/AIDS, Tuberculosis, and Malaria 22 USC Chapter 83.* Retrieved from uscode.house.gov/downloads/pls/23c82.txt.

Oinas, E., & Jungar, K. (2005, January). *No passive victims! Agents! The concept of victimhood in contemporary feminist debates, particularly in feminist HIV research.* Symposium conducted at the Writing African Women—Poetics and Politics of African Gender Research conference at the University of the Western Cape, Cape Town, South Africa.

One in Nine Campaign. (2012). *We were never meant to survive: Violence in the lives of HIV positive women.* Johannesburg, South Africa. Retrieved from http://www.oneinnine.org.za/58.page.

Oxfam International. (2007, February). *Oxfam calls for G7 to deliver for Africa.* Retrieved from http://www.oxfam.org/en/news/2007/pr070208_g7.

———. (2007, August). *Oxfam targeted with email campaign as Novartis' legal action against India approaches climax.* Retrieved from http://www.oxfam.org/en/news/2007/pr070215_novartis

PEPFAR. (2005). *The power of Partnerships: The President's Emergency Plan for AIDS Relief. 3rd annual report to Congress.* Retrieved from http://www.pepfar.gov/documents/organization/81019.pdf.

PEPFARWatch. (2008). *Abstinence and fidelity.* Retrieved August 15, 2012, from http://www.pepfarwatch.org/the_issues/abstinence_and_fidelity.

Persson, A. (2005). Facing HIV: Body shape change and the (in)visibility of illness. *Medical Anthropology, 24,* 237–264.

Petros, G., Airhihenbuwa, C. O., Simbayi, L., Ramlagan, S., & Brown, B. (2006). HIV/AIDS and "othering" in South Africa: The blame goes on. *Culture, Health & Sexuality, 8,* 67–77.

Petrus, T., & Isaacs-Martin, W. (2011). *The symbology of Colouredness: Meanings and interpretation of Coloured identity in South Africa.* Paper presented at 11th International Conference on Diversity in Organizations, Communities, and Nations. June 20–22.University of the Western Cape, Cape Town, South Africa.

Piot, P. (2001). A gendered epidemic: Women and the risks and burdens of HIV. *Journal of American Medical Women's Association, 56,* 609–611.

Pound, P., Britten, N., Morgan, M., Yardley, L., Pope, C., Daker-White, G., & Campbell, R. (2005). Resisting medicine: A synthesis of qualitative studies of medicine taking. *Social Science & Medicine, 62,* 133–155.

Preston-Whyte, E., Varga, C. Oosthuizen, H., Roberts, R., & Blose, F. (2000). Survival sex and HIV/AIDS in an African city. In R. Parker, R. M. Barbosa, & P. Aggleton (Eds.) *Framing the sexual subject: The politics of gender, sexuality, and power* (pp. 165–190). Berkeley, CA: University of California Press.

Provincial Administration Western Cape. (2004). *Antiretroviral treatment protocol.* Retrieved from http://web.uct.ac.za/depts/epi/artrollout.

Puoane, T., Fourie, J. M., Rosling, L., Tshaka, N. C., & Oelefse, A. (2005). "Big is beautiful"—An exploration with urban black community health workers in a South African township. *South African Journal of Clinical Nutrition, 18*(1), 8–15.

Puoane, T., Tsolekile, L., & Steyn, N. (2010). Perceptions about body image and sizes among Black African girls living in Cape Town. *Ethnicity and Disease, 20*(1), 29–34.

Raj, A., Silverman, J. G., & Amaro, H. (2004). Abused women report greater male partner risk and gender-based risk for HIV: Findings from a community-based study with Hispanic women. *AIDS Care, 16,* 519–530.

Ratele, K., & Shefer, T. (2002). Stigma in the social construction of sexually transmitted diseases. In D. Hook & G. Eagle (Eds.), *Psychopathology and Social Prejudice* (pp.185–206). Cape Town, South Africa: University of Cape Town Press.

Reddy, S. (2005). "It's not as easy as ABC": Dynamics of intergenerational power and resistance within the context of HIV. *Perspectives in Education, 23,* 11–19.

Reid, C., & Tom, A. (2006). Poor women's discourses of legitimacy, poverty and health. *Gender & Society, 20,* 402–421.

Reinharz, S. (1992). *Feminist methods in social research.* New York, NY: Oxford University Press.

Reischer, E., & Koo, K. S. (2004). The body beautiful: Symbolism and agency in the social world. *Annual Review of Anthropology, 33,* 297–317.

Reynolds, N. R., Neidig, J. L., Wu, A. W., Gifford, A. L., & Holmes, W. C. (2006). Balancing disfigurement and disease progression: Patient perceptions of HIV body fat distribution. *AIDS Care, 18,* 663–673.

Rhine, K. A. (2009). Support groups, marriage, and the management of ambiguity among HIV-positive women in northern Nigeria. *Anthropological Quarterly, 82*(2), 369–400.

Rivero-Mendez, M., Dawson-Rose, C. S., & Solis-Baez, S. S. (2010). A qualitative study of providers' perception of adherence of women living with HIV/AIDS in Puerto Rico. *Qualitative Report, 15*(2), 232–251.

Robins, S. (2006). From "rights" to "ritual": AIDS activism in South Africa. *American Anthropologist 108*(2), 312–323.

Rodin, J. (1993). Culture and psychosocial determinants of weight concerns. *Annals of Internal Medicine, 119,* 643–645.

Ross, R. (1994). *Beyond the pale: Essays on the history of colonial South Africa.* Johannesburg, South Africa: Witwatersrand University Press.

Rothenberg, K. R. (1995). Domestic violence and partner notification: Implications for treatment and counseling of women with HIV. *Journal of the American Medical Women Association, 50,* 87–93.

Salo, E. (2002). Condoms are for spares, not besties: Negotiating adolescent sexuality in post-apartheid Manenberg. *Society in Transition, 33*(3), 403–419.

———. (2005). Negotiating gender and personhood in the New South Africa: Adolescent women and gangsters in Manenberg Township on the Cape Flats. In S. Robins (Ed.), *Limits to Liberation* (pp. 173–189). London, England: James Currey.

———. (2006). *"We've got it covered"–what we know about condom use, personhood gender and generation across space in Cape Flats townships.* Address to World Library and Information Congress: 72nd IFLA General Conference and Council, 20–24 August 2006, Seoul, Korea.

Sample, I. (2010). Blanket HIV testing could see AIDS dying out in 40 years. *Guardian* February 21. Retrieved from http://www.guardian.co.uk/world/2010/feb/21 /blanket-testing-hiv-aids.

Scanlon, J. (1993). Challenging the imbalances of power in feminist oral history: Developing a take-and-give methodology. *Women's Studies International Forum, 16,* 649–645.

Schrimshaw, E. W., & Siegel, K. (2002). HIV-infected mothers' to their uninfected children: Rates, reasons, and reactions. *Journal of Social & Personal Relationships, 19,* 19–43.

Schwarzer, R., Dunkel-Schetter, C., & Kemeny, M. (1994). The multidimensional nature of received social support in gay men at risk of HIV infection and AIDS. *American Journal of Community Psychology, 22,* 319–339.

Seekings, J. (2008). The continuing salience of race: Discrimination and diversity in South Africa. *Journal of Contemporary African Studies, 26*(1), 1–25.

Seidel, G. (1993). The competing discourses of HIV/AIDS in sub-Saharan Africa: Discourses of rights and empowerment vs. discourses of control and exclusion. *Social Science & Medicine, 36*(3), 175–194.

Seidel, G., & Ntuli, N. (1996). HIV, confidentiality, gender, and support in rural South Africa. *Lancet, 347*(8999), 469–472.

Serovich, J. M. (2001). A test of two HIV disclosure theories. *AIDS Education Prevention, 13*(4), 355–364.

Serumaga-Zake, P., Kotze, D., & Madsen, R. (2005). A descriptive study of the dynamics of relative poverty in the Western Cape province of South Africa. *Development Southern Africa, 22*(1), 143–160.

Servellen, G. V., & Lombardi, E. (2005). Supportive relationships and medication adherence in HIV-infected low-income Latinos. *Western Journal of Nursing Research, 27,* 1023–1029.

Sessions, K. B. (2001). United States—The south. In R. A. Smith (Ed.), *Encyclopedia of AIDS: A social, political, culture, and scientific record of the HIV epidemic* (pp. 703–709). New York, NY: Penguin Books.

Sexuality Information and Education Council of the United States (SIECUS). (2009). *Making prevention work: Lessons from Zambia on reshaping the U.S. response to the global HIV/AIDS epidemic.* Retrieved from http://siecus.org/index.cfm?fuseaction=Feature.showFeature&FeatureID=1767.

Sharma, A., Howard, A. A., Klein, R. S., Schoenbaum, E. E., Buono, D., & Webber, M. P. (2007). Body image in older men with or at-risk for HIV infection. *AIDS Care, 19,* 235–241.

Shisana, O., Rehle, T., Simai, L. C., Zuma, K., Jooste, S., Pillay-van-Wyk, V., Mbelle, N. Van Zyl, P., Parker, W., Zungo, N. P., Pezi, S., & The SABSSM III Implementation Team. (2009). *South African National HIV prevalence, incidence, behaviour and communication survey, 2008: A turning tide among teenagers?* Cape Town, South Africa: HSRC Press. Retrieved from http://www.hsrcpress.ac.za/product.php?productid=2134.

Smith, D. J. (2009). Managing men, marriage and modern love: Women's perspectives on intimacy and male infidelity in southeastern Nigeria. In J. Cole & L. Thomas (Eds.) *Love in Africa* (pp. 157–180). Chicago, IL: University of Chicago Press.

Smitt, J., Middelkoop, K., Myer, L., Seedat, S., Wood, R., Stein, D. J., & Bekker, L. G. (2006). Sexual risk factors associated with volunteering for HIV vaccine research in South Africa. *AIDS Care, 18,* 569–573.

Sobo, E. J. (1994). The sweetness of fat: Health, procreation, and sociability in rural Jamaica. In N. Sault (Ed.), *Many mirrors: Body image and social relations* (pp. 132–152). New Brunswick, NJ: Rutgers University Press.

Southafrica.info. (2012). *A parent's guide to schooling.* Retrieved from http://www.southafrica.info/services/education/edufacts.htm.

Squire, C. (2007). *HIV in South Africa: Talking about the big thing.* London, England: Routledge.

Statistics South Africa. (2004). Home language. *Census 2001: Primary tables South Africa Census '96 and 2001 compared.* Retrieved from http://www.statssa.gov.za/census01/html/RSAPrimary.pdf.

———. (2011). *Midyear population estimates.* http://www.statssa.gov.za/publications/P0302/P03022011.pdf.

———. (2012). *Quarterly labour force survey: Quarter 1, 2012.* Retrieved from http://www.statssa.gov.za/publications/P0211/P02111stQuarter2012.pdf.

Steinberg, M., Johnson, S., Schierhout, G., & Ndegwa, D. (2002). *Hitting home: How households cope with the impact of the HIV/AIDS epidemic. A survey of households affected by HIV/AIDS in South Africa.* Washington DC: Henry J. Kaiser Family Foundation.

Strebel, A. (1995). Whose epidemic is it? Reviewing the literature on women and AIDS. *South African Journal of Psychology, 25,* 12–20.

Summers, J., Robinson, R., Capps, L., Zisook, S., Atkinson, J. H., McCutchan, E., McCutchan, J. A., Deutsch, R., Patterson, T., & Grant, I. (2000). The influence of HIV-related support groups on survival in women who lived with HIV. *Psychosomatics, 41* (3), 262–266.

Swartz, L., & Kagee, A. (2006). Community participation in AIDS vaccine trials: Empowerment or science. *Social Science and Medicine, 63,* 1143–1146.

TAC (Treatment Action Campaign). (2007, April). *APL submissions to human rights commission enquiry into access to health care services.* Retrieved from http://tac.org.za/documents/ALPsubmissionSAHRChearingsonhealth170407.pdf.

TAC.org.za. (2012). http://www.tac.org.za/community.

Taliep, W. (2001). Belletjiesbos, Draper Street and the Vlak: The Coloured neighbourhoods of Claremont before group areas. *African Studies, 60*(1), 65–85.

Taylor, M., Kelvin Mwaba, N., & Rule, C. (2011). *Coloured identity in post-apartheid South Africa: A study of the new experience of personhood.* Paper presented at 11th International Conference on Diversity in Organizations, Communities, and Nations. June 20–22. University of the Western Cape, Cape Town, South Africa.

Temmerman, M. (1995). The right not to know HIV test results. *Lancet, 345,* 969–970.

Terre Blanche, M., Durrheim, K., & Painter, D. (1999). *Research in practice: Applied methods for the social sciences.* Cape Town, South Africa: Juta Academic.

———. (2006). *Research in practice: Applied methods for the social sciences.* Cape Town, South Africa: University of Cape Town Press.

Theorell T., Blomkvist, V., Jonsson, H., Schulman, S., Berntorp, E., & Stigendal, L. (1995). Social support and the development of immune function in human immunodeficiency virus infection. *Psychosomatic Medicine, 57,* 32–36.

Tiessen, R. (2005). Mainstreaming gender in HIV/AIDS programs: Ongoing challenges and new opportunities in Malawi. *Journal of International Women's Studies, 7,* 8–25.

Tong, R. (2009). *Feminist thought: A more comprehensive introduction.* Boulder, CO: Westview Press.

Tostes, M. A., Chalub, M., & Botega, N. J. (2004). The quality of life of HIV-infected women is associated with psychiatric morbidity. *AIDS Care, 16*, 177–187.

True, J. (2003). Mainstreaming gender in global public policy. *International Feminist Journal of Politics, 5*, 368–396.

UNAIDS. (2008). *2008 Report on the global AIDS epidemic.* Retrieved from http://www .unaids.org/en/dataanalysis/knowyourepidemic/epidemiologypublications /2008reportontheglobalaidsepidemic.

———. (2010). *UNAIDS report on the global AIDS epidemic.* Retrieved from http://www .unaids.org/globalreport/Global_report.htm.

———. (2011). *World AIDS Day report.* Retrieved from http://www.unaids.org/en/media /unaids/contentassets/documents/factsheet/2011/20111121_FS_WAD2011_global _en.pdf.

———. (2012a). *Report on the global AIDS epidemic.* Retrieved from http://www.unaids .org/en/dataanalysis/knowyourresponse/countryprogressreports/2012countries.

———. (2012b). *UNAIDS regional factsheet 2012.* Retrieved from http://www.unaids.org /en/media/unaids/contentassets/documents/epidemiology/2012/gr2012/2012_FS _regional_ssa_en.pdf

UNAIDS/UNFPA/UNIFEM (2004). *Women and HIV/AIDS: Confronting the crisis.* Retrieved from http://www.unfpa.org/upload/lib_pub_file/308_filename_women _aids1.pdf.

UNICEF (2006). *Africa's orphaned generations.* Retrieved from http://www.unicef.org /sowc06/pdfs/africas_orphans.pdf.

UN Women. (2012). *Effective approaches to addressing the intersection of violence against women and HIV/AIDS: Findings from programmes supported by the UN trust fund to end violence against women.* Retrieved from http://www.unwomen .org/wp-content/uploads/2012/04/ UNTF_2012_ VAW-and-HIV.pdf.

Urdang, S. (2006). The care economy: Gender and the silent AIDS crisis in southern Africa. *Journal of Southern African Studies, 32*, 166–177.

Van der Straten, A., King, R., Grinstead, O., Serufilira, A., & Allen, S. (1995). Couple communication, sexual coercion and HIV risk reduction in Kigali, Rwanda. *AIDS, 9*, 935–944.

Visser, M. J., Makin, J. D., & Lehobye, K. (2006). Stigmatising attitudes of the community towards people living with HIV. *Journal of Community & Applied Social Psychology, 16*, 42–58.

Visser, M. J., & Mundell, J. P. (2008). Establishing support groups for HIV-infected women: Using experiences to develop guiding principles for project implementation. *Journal of Social Aspects of HIV/AIDS/Journal de Aspects Sociaux du VIH/ SIDA, 5*(2), 65–73.

Weitz, R. (2010). A history of women's bodies. In R. Weitz (Ed.) *The politics of women's bodies: Sexuality, appearance and behavior* (pp. 3–12). New York, NY: Oxford University Press.

Whittaker, A. M. (1992). Living with HIV: Resistance by positive people. *Medical Anthropology Quarterly, 6*, 385–390.

Wilson, D., Naidoo, S., Bekker, L. G., Cotton, M., & Maartens, G. (2004). *Oxford handbook of HIV medicine.* Cape Town, South Africa: Oxford University Press Southern Africa.

Wiss, R. (1994). Lipreading: Remembering Saartjie Baartman. *Australian Journal of Anthropology,* 5, 11–40.

Wodak, W., & Meyer, M. (2001). *Methods of Critical Discourse Analysis.* London, England: Sage Publications.

Wolf, D. L. (Ed.). (1996). Feminist dilemmas in field work. Boulder, CO: Westview Press.

Wood, S. A., Tobias, C., & McCree, J. (2004). Medication adherence for HIV positive women caring for children: In their own words. *AIDS Care,* 16, 909–913.

Worden, N. (1985). *Slavery in Dutch South Africa.* Cambridge, UK: Cambridge University Press.

Yalom, I. D. (1995). *The theory and practice of group psychotherapy* (4th ed.). New York, NY: Basic Books.

Zegeye, A. (2002). A matter of colour. *African and Asian Studies,* 1(4), 323–348.

Zeleza, P. T. (2002, July). *Rethinking Africa's gender and globalisation dynamics.* Paper presented at the Women's Worlds Congress, 8th International Interdisciplinary Congress on Women, Makerere University, Kampala, Uganda.

Contributors

Anna Aulette-Root is a PhD candidate at the University of Cape Town, where she lectures in psychology. She holds a Master of Social Science degree in psychology from UCT and is a member of the Men, Masculinities & Violence research project in the department. Her current research interests are in the areas of critical feminism, qualitative methodology, intersectionality theory, femininities and masculinities, HIV, and social action and activism. Her dissertation is based on the life stories of men who have been violent toward intimate partners in Cape Town. She especially enjoys teaching undergraduate as well as graduate students at UCT and strives to spark their interest in pursuing research and careers in areas that will contribute toward social change.

Floretta Boonzaier is Senior Lecturer in the Department of Psychology at the University of Cape Town. Her primary research areas include psychological aspects of gender-based violence; the intersections of raced, classed, and gendered subjectivities; and a focus on the social construction of femininities and masculinities in the postapartheid South African context. She has published on intimate partner violence against women locally and internationally. In 2009 she was awarded the UCT Mandela Fellowship at the W. E. B. Du Bois Institute for African and African American Research at Harvard University. In 2010 she received the runner-up award in the Department of Science and Technology's Women in Science awards, for the category of Distinguished Young Woman Researcher in the Social Sciences or Humanities.

Judy Aulette is Professor in the Department of Sociology and the Women's and Gender Studies Program at the University of North Carolina–Charlotte, where she teaches courses in gender, family, race ethnicity, and qualitative methods. In addition, she currently teaches a distance education course for the University of the Western Cape in Cape Town. She has published books and articles on gender, families, women in Cape Verde, and women and social activism. Her latest project is on South-South migration, exploring the experience of women care workers who have migrated from the Philippines and Ethiopia to work in Iraq. She is the recipient of two Fulbright awards to South Africa and Poland and has taught at a number of universities in Europe.

Index

CPSIA information can be obtained at www.ICGtesting.com
Printed in the USA
BVOW08s1031050214

344033BV00003B/40/P